Exercise in Water

Every physiotherapist in training and practice today needs a knowledge and experience of pool therapy. *Exercise in Water*, which covers the requirements of the Syllabus, provides a lucid explanation of the physical properties of water and its physiological and therapeutic effects. By providing a true understanding of the properties of water this book will enable the physiotherapist to adapt her basic training to the special requirements of the new medium. Progressive exercises are described and illustrated and are easily adaptable to individual needs and circumstances.

There are special chapters on the treatment of rheumatic, neurological and orthopaedic conditions, and the lively and imaginative chapter on the treatment of children will be welcomed by the therapist who has young patients in her care.

This book is dedicated to Mary Ainsworth
who did so much to encourage and inspire others
to further their knowledge of hydrotherapy

Exercise in Water

EDITED BY

M. H. DUFFIELD, M.C.S.P., Dip.P.T.

Principal, School of Physiotherapy
The Middlesex Hospital, London

LONDON
BAILLIÈRE, TINDALL AND CASSELL

First published 1969

© 1969 Baillière, Tindall & Cassell Ltd
7 and 8 Henrietta Street, London WC2

SBN 7020 0303 4

Published in the United States by
The Williams & Wilkins Company, Baltimore

Printed in Great Britain by
William Clowes and Sons, Limited, London and Beccles

Contributors

Dr A. C. Boyle, M.B., B.S., D.Phys. Med., M.D., F.R.C.P.
Physician-in-Charge, Department of Physical Medicine and Rheumatism, The Middlesex Hospital, London

Miss A. E. Bartholomew, F.C.S.P.
Superintendent Physiotherapist, The Middlesex Hospital, London

Miss M. H. Duffield, M.C.S.P., Dip.P.T.
Principal, School of Physiotherapy, The Middlesex Hospital, London

Miss C. H. Gilmore, M.C.S.P., H.T.
Lecturer, School of Physiotherapy, Royal Prince Alfred Hospital, Sydney, New South Wales (1967) and University of Queensland (1968). Formerly Physiotherapist, The Middlesex Hospital, London

Mrs M. J. Reid, M.C.S.P.
Deputy Superintendent, Great Ormond Street Hospital for Sick Children, London. Formerly Superintendent Physiotherapist, Franklin Delano Roosevelt School for Physically Handicapped Children, London

Mrs Y. M. Rogers (née Harrison), M.C.S.P., H.T.
Physiotherapist, The Middlesex Hospital, London

Mrs J. O. Shipley (née Berry), M.C.S.P., H.T.
Senior Physiotherapist-in-Charge, Hydrotherapy Unit, The Middlesex Hospital, London

Miss A. T. Skinner, M.C.S.P., H.T., Dip.P.T.
Teacher, School of Physiotherapy, The Middlesex Hospital, London

Contents

Preface   ix

Introduction   1

1. Basic Physics and their Application   4
2. The Physiological and Therapeutic Effects
   of Exercise in Warm Water   21
3. Theory of Treatments   26
4. Dangers and Precautions   42
5. Pools, Tanks and Accessory Equipment   48
6. Indications and Contra-indications   58
7. The Treatment of Rheumatic Disorders   61
8. The Treatment of Neurological Disorders   71
9. The Treatment of Orthopaedic Conditions   88
10. Children in Water   112

Index   121

Plates

Between pages

I, II. The Pack   54–55

III. A Sunken Pool

IV. The Pool at St Benedict's Hospital,
    London

V. The Hubbard Tank

VI. An Electrically Operated Hoist

VII. Accessory Apparatus

VIII. Float Lying

Preface

WHEN the Chartered Society of Physiotherapy's revised syllabus came into operation at the beginning of 1965, pool therapy became a compulsory subject for every student in training. As a result of this it is now being widely taught and all students qualifying will know the basic principles. Many physiotherapists who qualified before this date will not have received this training and, as many more pools are now being installed, are finding themselves at a disadvantage. It is hoped that this book will not only prove useful to students in training but also to qualified physiotherapists who are carrying out pool treatments.

The chapter on Children in Water owes much to the advice and experience of Mr J. McMillan, honorary secretary of the Association of Swimming Therapy, and I would like to thank him for all the help he gave when this chapter was being written. Acknowledgement is also due to Dr M. D. Wilson, inspector for special education to the Inner London Education Authority. Plates IV and V were first published in *Physiotherapy* and are reproduced by permission of the Editor.

I would like to thank all the contributors for their patience and forbearance during the compiling of this book, and Mrs R. J. Clarke for correcting the proofs.

August 1969   M. H. DUFFIELD

Introduction

THE term hydrotherapy is derived from the Greek words *hydor*—water, and *therapeia*—healing. There is no very clear evidence as to when water was first used for healing purposes but it is known that Hippocrates (*c.* 460–*c.* 375 B.C.) used hot and cold water (contrast baths) in the treatment of disease. Water for recreational and curative purposes was used widely by the Romans. They had four types of bath of varying temperature: the frigidarium was a cold bath and was used only for recreational purposes; the tepidarium consisted of a tepid bath sited in a room containing warm air; the caldarium contained a hot bath and the sudatonium was a room filled with moist hot air to promote sweating. The remains of these baths may still be seen at Bath and Buxton and many other places both in this country and abroad.

Little more was heard of this method of treatment until 1697 when Sir John Flayer, a physician living in Lichfield, published a paper on 'An Enquiry into the Right Use and Abuse of Hot, Cold and Temperate Baths in England'. He followed this twenty-five years later with a 'History of Cold Bathing'. He advocated that hot baths should be used in hot countries and cold baths in cold countries, but he himself opened a centre for tepid baths in Lichfield. In spite of dedicating his second paper to the Royal College of Physicians his teaching received little support in England, although in Germany tepid baths were used extensively for the relief of muscle spasm and in the treatment of hyper-excitable patients.

In 1779 a ship's surgeon, Doctor Wright, published his findings on the use of cold in the treatment of smallpox, and subsequently he used this form of treatment for many febrile conditions at a clinic he opened in Edinburgh. He stimulated Doctor Currie, a Liverpool physician, to investigate further the effects produced by cold, and he published a paper on 'Medical Reports of the Effect of Water, Cold and Warm, as a Remedy for Fever'. He advocated the 'subtraction of heat' for sedation of the nervous system. Although Currie's methods were used widely on the Continent, they did not find favour with the medical profession in England.

In 1830 a Silesian peasant, Vincent Pressnitz, set up a centre for the use of cold water and vigorous exercise. These methods did receive some support in this country, but centres which were opened in Matlock and Malvern did not survive for long as they were used chiefly by unqualified practitioners and were looked down on by the medical profession. However, Pressnitz stimulated considerable thought on the Continent and for the first time scientific investigation was undertaken into the reactions of the tissues to water at various temperatures, and their reaction in disease. Taking part in these investigations was Doctor Winterwitz of Vienna, who made a further study of the works of Wright and Currie, finally establishing an accepted physiological basis for hydrotherapy.

As in this country, there was considerable opposition at first to the therapeutic use of water in France, Italy and America but gradually it gained favour in these countries and treatment centres were established in all of them, although it was not until 1903 that the first centre was opened in the United States, in Boston.

Like many other forms of treatment, the use of hydrotherapy met with suspicion at first, partly because unsupported and extravagant claims were made for its effects and value. Gradually, however, it became accepted as a recognized form of treatment for nervous and other disorders. It is interesting to note that early emphasis was laid on the use of cold, and today ice has become an increasingly popular form of treatment for, among other conditions, the relief of muscle spasm.

At the beginning of this century treatment in the spas in this country was given by people with little training or medical knowledge and it was available only to those members of the community who could afford to visit them. The many physicians who specialized in the treatment of rheumatism felt that this was unsatisfactory, and largely at their instigation the British Red Cross Society opened a clinic for the treatment of Rheumatic Diseases at Peto Place in London. It was formally opened by Her Majesty Queen Mary in 1930 and it was staffed by chartered physiotherapists with Miss McAllister, s.r.n., c.s.m.m.g., in charge. The Council of the Chartered Society then approved a syllabus for a post-registration training in hydrotherapy to be taken at this clinic. This was quickly superseded by a longer twelve-week course followed by an examination. Soon after this, a similar training course was started in Cardiff and later in Bath, Buxton and Harrogate. With some modifications this training has continued to the present day, but recently it was decided that the principles of pool therapy should be included in the three-year course for physiotherapists and the post-registration courses as such have ceased to exist.

I

Basic Physics and their Application

IN ORDER TO UNDERSTAND the principles of hydrotherapy it is necessary to acquire a knowledge of the physical properties of water, particularly in their relation to the concepts of matter.

Matter. Anything that occupies space is known as matter. It is composed of molecules which, in turn, are composed of atoms. All matter exists in three forms: as solids, liquids or gases. Water is an example of a substance which can exist in any of the three states—ice, water and steam. Below 0°C (32°F) water is solid, between 0°C (32°F) and 100°C (212°F) it is liquid, and above 100°C (212°F), gaseous.

PHYSICAL PROPERTIES OF WATER

In common with other forms of matter, water has certain physical properties which include: (1) mass, (2) weight, (3) density, (4) specific gravity, (5) buoyancy, (6) hydrostatic pressure, (7) surface tension, (8) refraction and (9) viscosity.

1. MASS

The mass of a substance is the amount of material it comprises.

2. WEIGHT

The weight of a substance is the force with which it is attracted towards the centre of the earth.

Relationship between mass and weight. Mass is unalterable and is measured in pounds or grams. Weight is the effect of gravity upon the mass, and alters according to the position of a body in relation to the earth. Units of measurement are poundals in the F.P.S. system or dynes in the C.G.S. system. A poundal is the force which, acting on 1 lb matter for 1 sec, generates a velocity of 1 ft per sec; and a dyne is the force which, acting on a mass of 1 g for 1 sec, generates a velocity of 1 cm/per sec.

$$W = Mg$$

where W = weight, M = mass and g = force of gravity. The force of gravity is approximately 981 cm/sec² (32 ft/sec²).

A mass of 1 lb (0·45 kg), therefore, has a weight of 32 poundals, and a mass of 1 gram, a weight of 981 dynes.* For everyday purposes, however, the weight of a body is compared with the standard pound weight which is a cylinder of platinum kept at the Board of Trade Standard Office. Thus a body with a mass of 1 lb is said to weigh 1 lb because it balances the standard pound weight on a pair of scales.

Weight (mass) of water = 10 lb per gallon at 4°C (39·2°F)

3. DENSITY

A wooden log weighing a ton will float but an iron nail weighing a few ounces will sink; this is because wood is less dense than iron.

The density of a substance is the relationship between the mass and volume of a substance.

$$Density = \frac{Mass}{Volume}$$

Mass per unit volume is expressed as grams per cubic centimetre (cm³). Water is most dense at 4°C (39·2°F). It expands at both higher and lower temperatures and therefore ice is less dense than water and floats (Fig. 1). The density of ice is 0·92 g/cm³, that of iron 7·7 g/cm³, and that of wood is 0·75 g/cm³; the average density of the human body is 0·95 g/cm³. Dissolved substances increase the density of water; therefore, sea water for example is denser (1·024 g/cm³) than fresh water (1 g/cm³).

4. SPECIFIC GRAVITY

The specific gravity or relative density of a substance is the ratio of the mass of a given volume of the substance to the mass of the same volume of water. The specific gravity of water is 1; a

* The dyne and poundal are replaced by the newton (N) in the Système International d'Unités (SI) which is now being widely adopted in many countries including Britain. The newton is the force which acting on a mass of 1 kg for 1 sec generates a velocity of 1 m per sec.

body with a specific gravity of less than 1 will float, and a body
with more than 1 will sink in water.

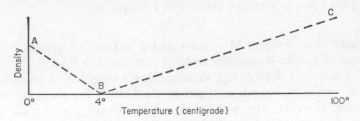

Fig. 1. Change in density of water with temperature variation. (Broken
line shows the expansion of water)

5. BUOYANCY

Of the physical laws of water that the hydrotherapist should
understand, and apply when giving pool therapy, those of buoyancy
(Archimedes' principle), and of hydrostatic pressure are most
important.

Archimedes' Principle. The principle of Archimedes states that
when a body is wholly or partially immersed in a fluid at rest it
experiences an upthrust equal to the weight of fluid displaced.
Therefore, if a body has a specific gravity of less than 1 it will float,
since the weight of the object is less than the weight of water displaced. If the specific gravity is greater than 1 it will sink, and if
equal to 1 it will float just below the surface of the water.

Since the average specific gravity of the human body with air in
the lungs is 0·95, it will float. When the body is floating the ratio
of the submerged parts to those which are not submerged is
0·95:0·05. If the submerged portion of the body exceeds 0·05, as
when a person has the head and arms fixed above the water level,
the amount of water displaced by the remainder will be insufficient
to support the weight of the body and the pelvis and legs will sink.
However, if a support such as a float is placed round the pelvis,
the lower part of the body will not sink (Figs 2–4).

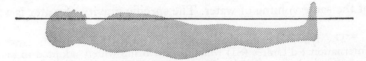

Fig. 2. Body floating at rest

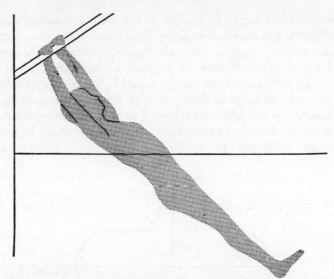

Fig. 3. Insufficient water displacement

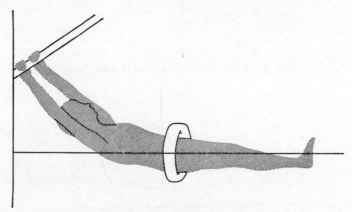

Fig. 4. Use of pelvic float

A submarine can submerge or float at will because its density can be altered by increasing or decreasing the proportion of air to water in the ballast tanks. Similarly, in the human body, the density can be altered by increasing or decreasing the amount of air in the lungs. Hence a person whose lungs are filled with air on inspiration will float, but he will sink when he breathes out on expiration.

2

As wood has a specific gravity of less than 1, wooden sticks or crutches used in the pool must be made more dense than water by adding weights at their ends; alternatively, they can be made of solid metal. The amount of support or resistance given to a patient by inflatable floats can be varied by increasing or decreasing the amount of air in them, thereby altering their density.

Buoyancy is the force experienced as an upthrust which acts in the opposite direction to the force of gravity. A body in water is therefore subjected to two opposing forces—gravity, acting

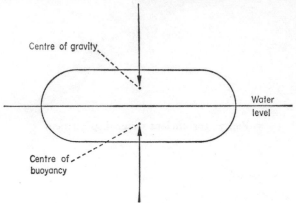

Fig. 5. A floating body in stable equilibrium

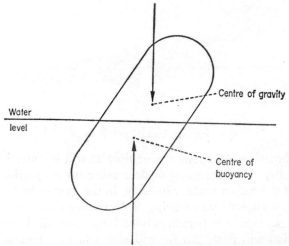

Fig. 6. Interaction of gravity and buoyancy

through the centre of gravity, and buoyancy, acting through the centre of buoyancy which is the centre of gravity of the displaced liquid. When the weight of the floating body equals the weight of the liquid displaced, and the centres of buoyancy and gravity are in the same vertical line, the body is kept in stable equilibrium. If the centres are not in the same vertical line the two forces acting on the body will cause it to roll over until it reaches a position of stable equilibrium (Figs 5, 6).

Moment of force. The moment of force about a point is the turning effect of the force about that point. As buoyancy is itself a force, this rule will govern its action.

Moment of buoyancy. This is represented by

$$F \times d$$

where F = the force of buoyancy, d = the perpendicular distance from a vertical line through A to the centre of buoyancy, and A = the point about which the turning effect of buoyancy is exerted.

Figure 7 illustrates this principle by showing the force of

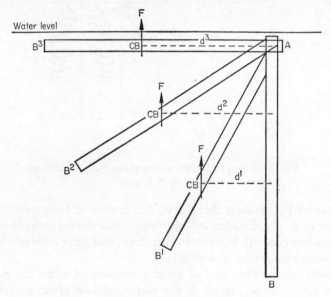

Fig. 7. The turning effect of buoyancy
A lever (A–B) is submerged in water. F = force of
buoyancy; CB = centre of buoyancy; d = distance
from vertical

buoyancy and the centre of buoyancy on a lever submerged in
water at three different angles. The moment of buoyancy on
$$AB^1 = F \times d^1$$
and on $\qquad\qquad AB^2 = F \times d^2.$

As d^2 is greater than d^1 the moment of force is greater on AB^2 than
on AB^1. In the vertical position $d = $ zero, so there is no turning
effect, but as the lever comes to the surface the effect is increased
and is maximal at B^3 where d^3 is greatest.

In the human body the lever is formed by the limbs, A being
the joint about which movement is occurring. When A represents
the shoulder joint, and the upper extremity is AB, the moment of
force, i.e. the turning effect of buoyancy, increases with the degree
of abduction. The effect of buoyancy therefore increases as the
limb approaches the surface of the water (Fig. 8). If the lever is

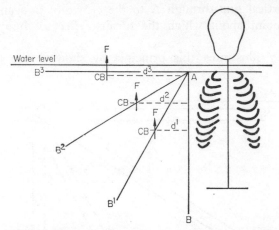

Fig. 8. Effect of buoyancy increasing on abduction
Key as in Fig. 7

shortened by bending the elbow, the centre of buoyancy moves
nearer to A, the distance d is shortened and the moment of buoyancy is less (Fig. 9). Buoyancy, therefore, will have a greater effect
on a long rather than a short lever.

Buoyancy may be used to assist a movement when the part is
taken towards the surface of the water, and to resist movement
when the part is taken from the surface of the water to the
vertical position. The moment of buoyancy increases (a) as the
limb moves nearer to the surface of the water, and (b) as the lever

lengthens. Therefore, when re-educating weak muscles, a longer lever and an inner range movement gain the most assistance from buoyancy. However, when the movement is carried out against the force of buoyancy, there will be resistance to the movement which lessens (a) as the limb nears the vertical position, and (b) with a shorter lever. The maximum resistance of buoyancy is thus exerted on a long lever near to the outer range of movement.

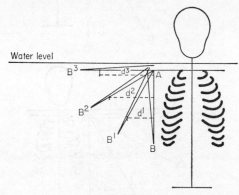

Fig. 9. A weaker effect due to bending the elbow
Key as in Fig. 7

The assistance or resistance of buoyancy can be increased still further by using floats which alter the position of the centre of buoyancy, and so the distance between the centre and the point about which the force of buoyancy exerts its turning effect. (In Fig. 10(a) d is shorter than in Fig. 10(b), and so the moment of force has increased.)

When a person stands almost upright in water his body tends to return to the vertical position, but during walking or sitting the legs tend to be displaced to the surface if they are raised too high and the body overbalances backwards (Figs 11, 12). The 'weight relief' of the body due to the upthrust of buoyancy is one of the main advantages of pool treatment.

6. HYDROSTATIC PRESSURE

The molecules of a fluid thrust upon each part of the surface area of an immersed body. This thrust per unit area is the pressure of the fluid. Pascal's Law states that fluid pressure is exerted equally on all surface areas of an immersed body at rest at a given

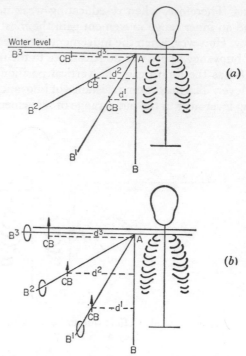

Fig. 10. Effect of buoyancy altered by addition of float

depth (Fig. 13). Pressure increases (a) with the density of the fluid, and (b) with its depth. For example, the pressure exerted by alcohol is less than that of water and the pressure exerted by sea water is more than that of fresh water at a given depth.

The pressure of the water is felt when a person enters the pool. It is most evident on the chest, where the water resists expansion, so it is usually inadvisable to put patients with a vital capacity of less than 1500 cm³ into a pool. Due to the pressure of the water which may be 488·24 kg/m² care should be taken when treating weak patients. Being equal in all directions, the pressure is not felt more on one surface of the body than another, and will give uniform resistance at a given depth. As pressure increases with depth, swelling will be reduced more easily if exercises are given well below the surface of the water where the increased pressure may be used. The lateral pressure exerted and the effect of buoyancy together will give the feeling of weightlessness.

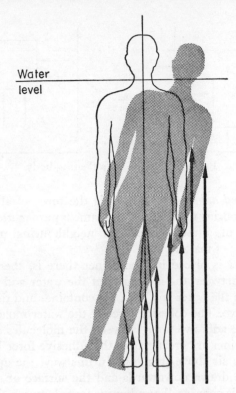

Water
level

Force of buoyancy

Fig. 11. Temporary displacement of vertical body

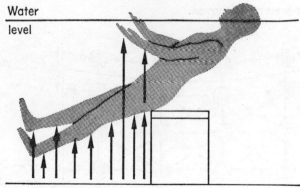

Water
level

Force of buoyancy

Fig. 12. Displacement during activity

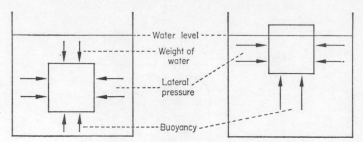

Fig. 13. Pressure on a floating body

Cohesion and adhesion. Cohesion is the force of attraction between neighbouring molecules of the same type of matter. Adhesion is the force of attraction between neighbouring molecules of different types of matter.

When water is placed in a container there is, therefore, a cohesive force between the molecules of the water and an adhesive force between the water and both the container and the molecules of the air above. The cohesive force of the water molecules themselves and the adhesive force between the molecules of the water and the container are greater than the adhesive force between the water and the air above (Fig. 14). In this way, the upper surface molecules arc drawn downwards and the surface of the water in the container is concave. The adhesive force between the container and the water molecules is greater than the cohesive force of the water, and this results in the walls of the container remaining wet after the water is removed.

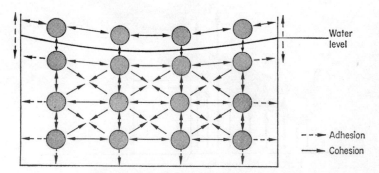

Fig. 14. Cohesive and adhesive forces

7. SURFACE TENSION

This is the force exerted between the surface molecules of a fluid. The force is probably due to cohesion between the molecules and manifests itself as an elastic 'skin' at the surface of the fluid. The tendency is thus for the area at the surface to try to contract to a minimum. The surface tension of water can be demonstrated by floating a needle on the surface of the water.

Surface tension acts as a resistance to movement when a limb is partially submerged as the surface tension has to be broken by the movement. Exercises can be made more difficult by utilizing surface tension; for example, an exercise is more difficult to perform on the surface than it is just below the surface where the surface tension does not have to be broken, but the effect is small.

8. REFRACTION

This is the bending of a ray as it passes from a more to a less dense medium or vice versa. When a ray passes from a rarer to a denser medium as from air to water, it bends towards the normal; passage in the opposite direction, from a denser to a rarer medium, bends the ray away from the normal. The normal is a line at right angles to the surface of the water (Figs 15, 16).

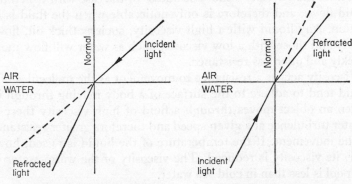

Fig. 15. Bending of light
towards normal

Fig. 16. Bending of light
away from normal

Let us consider a ray of light reflected from the bottom of the pool. The ray will be refracted away from the normal as it passes from the water to the air, hence point A appears to occur at point B because the observer assumes that light travels only in a straight line. The pool, therefore, seems to be shallower than it is (Fig. 17). The patient's limbs appear distorted, those partially submerged seeming to be bent away from the normal at water level. This means that movement of the joints may be difficult to determine.

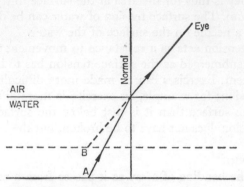

Fig. 17. The effect of light on the apparent bottom of pool
A = true bottom; B = false bottom

9. VISCOSITY

This is the type of friction that occurs between the molecules of a liquid and causes a resistance to flow of the liquid. Such friction expresses the viscosity—the 'stickiness' or the ease with which the liquid flows, and therefore is only noticeable when the fluid is in motion. Any liquid with a high viscosity, such as thick oil, flows slowly and those with a low viscosity such as water will flow more quickly and offer less resistance.

Viscosity acts as a resistance to movement as the molecules of a liquid tend to adhere to the surface of a body moving through it. When an object moves through a fluid of high viscosity there is greater turbulence at a given speed and therefore greater resistance to the movement. If the temperature of the liquid is raised, however, its viscosity is reduced. The viscosity of the warm water in the pool is less than in cold sea water.

Movement through water

The behaviour of a fluid is controlled by the nature and rate of flow. Professor Osborne Reynolds (1849–1912) proved that the flow of a liquid may be either streamlined or turbulent. He injected dye at constant velocity into a stream of fluid and found that when the fluid flowed slowly the dye appeared as a thread in the stream (streamline or laminar) flow, but when the flow was increased the dye twisted and eventually mixed completely with the fluid (turbulent flow). Turbulent flow is produced when the velocity of flow is increased beyond a certain level—the *critical velocity*. Liquids of a high viscosity have a high critical velocity.

Streamline flow is a continuous steady movement of fluid, the rate of movement at any fixed point remaining constant. It can be pictured as very thin layers of fluid molecules sliding over one another, the inner layers moving quickly, the outer ones moving slowly, and the outermost ones remaining stationary (Fig. 18).

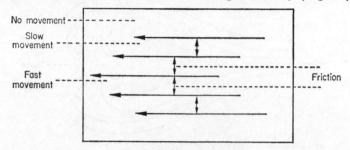

Fig. 18. Streamline flow

Turbulent flow is an irregular movement of the fluid, the movement varying at any fixed point (Fig. 19). This type of flow creates occasional rotary movements called eddies. It can be visualized as rapid, random movements of fluid molecules.

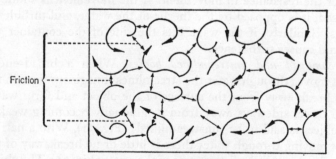

Fig. 19. Turbulent flow

Frictional resistance due to turbulent flow is greater than that due to streamline flow. In streamline flow resistance is directly proportional to velocity, while in turbulent flow resistance is proportional to the square of the velocity. The resistance offered by streamline flow is due to friction between layers of the fluid molecules only, whereas in turbulent flow the resistance is due to friction both between individual fluid molecules (as opposed to layers), and between the fluid and the container surface.

When an object moves through water, difference in water pressure develops between the front and the back of the object. The pressure builds up in front and decreases at the rear, resulting in a flow of water into the area of reduced pressure—known as 'the wake' (Fig. 20). Eddies form in the wake, partly from the water

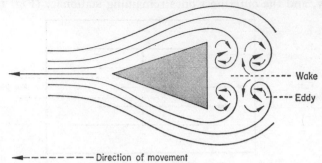

Fig. 20. Formation of wake and eddies

round the edges, and partly from the water behind the object. Flow in the wake is thus impeded, tending to drag the object back. The faster the movement, the greater is the drag, and therefore the greater the resistance to movement. If the movement is suddenly reversed, it is opposed by the inertia of the water, and turbulence occurs. Similarly, if the wake hits the side of the container the rebound causes turbulence.

Streamlined and unstreamlined bodies. When a broad-ended object moves through water the streamlines (imaginary lines in the fluid) break away from the surface of the object and form waves which travel sideways away from it, gradually becoming weaker. The object is said to be 'unstreamlined' (Fig. 21). With a narrow object moving through water there is little or no breakaway of the streamlines, and little disturbance of the water (Fig. 22). The object is said to be 'streamlined'. With an unstreamlined body there is greater wave formation and so greater resistance to its movement.

Practical applications of turbulence:

1. Turbulence can be used as a form of resistance to exercises

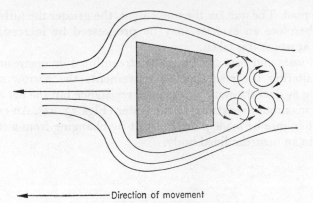

Direction of movement

Fig. 21. Unstreamlined object

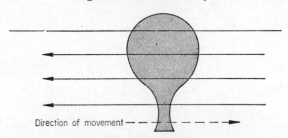

Direction of movement

Fig. 22. Streamlined object

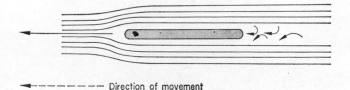

Direction of movement

Fig. 23. Streamlined flow across surface of bat

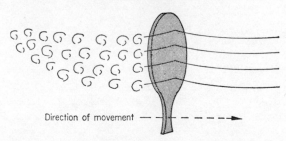

Direction of movement

Fig. 24. Bat facing flow of water causing turbulence

in the pool. The quicker the movement, the greater the turbulence and therefore an exercise may be progressed by increasing the speed at which it is taken.

2. Floats and bats can be made streamlined or unstreamlined, thus altering the resistance to movement: the narrow surface moving against the water offers little resistance but the flat surface offers maximum resistance to the water (Figs 23, 24). An exercise may therefore be made more difficult by changing from a streamlined to an unstreamlined body.

2

The Physiological and Therapeutic Effects of Exercise in Warm Water

THE physiological effects of pool therapy combine those brought about by the hot water of the pool with those of exercise, but the extent of such effects varies with the temperature of the water, the length of the treatment and the type and severity of the exercise. The average temperature of the water in the pool is 35·5°–36·6°C (96°–98°F) and the immersion period for most patients is 20 minutes, although some patients may begin with as little as 5 minutes or may stay in for as long as 45 minutes.

PHYSIOLOGICAL EFFECTS

DURING IMMERSION

During the period of immersion the physiological effects are similar to those brought about by any other form of heat but are less localized. A general rise in body temperature frequently occurs owing to several factors. The temperature of the water is above that of skin temperature, which is normally 33·5°C (92°–93°F). The body therefore gains heat through the areas under water but can lose it only from the blood in the cutaneous vessels and the sweat glands of the exposed areas, such as the face and neck. The body gains heat not only from the water, but also from all the contracting muscles performing the exercises. A rise in body temperature is therefore inevitable, the rise varying from patient to patient 37·5°C (99°F) or more.

As the skin becomes heated the superficial blood vessels dilate and the peripheral blood supply is increased. The blood flowing through these vessels is heated and, by convection, the temperature of the underlying structures (such as muscles) rises, their vessels dilate and their blood supply increases. This results in a redistribution of blood and the splanchnic vessels constrict to supply the increased volume of blood to the periphery. The heart rate increases with the temperature rise and as a result of exercise, the increase being proportional to the temperature of the water and the severity of the exercise.

As the patient enters the pool the cutaneous vessels constrict momentarily, causing a rise in peripheral resistance and a momentary rise in blood pressure. During immersion the arterioles dilate, therefore both the peripheral resistance and the blood pressure will fall.

A rise in temperature increases metabolism, therefore metabolism in the skin and muscles is increased and, as the body temperature rises, so does the general metabolic rate. This increases not only the demand for oxygen but also the production of carbon dioxide, causing the respiratory rate to increase in proportion.

The relatively mild heat of the water reduces the sensitivity of sensory nerve endings, and as the muscles are warmed by the blood passing through them their tone will diminish.

AFTER IMMERSION

When the patient leaves the pool the heat loss mechanism comes into operation and the temperature returns to normal, owing chiefly to the considerable activity of the sweat glands; this results in considerable fluid loss from the body. Immediately after treatment the patient rests in a pack which restricts heat loss from the surface capillaries but encourages sweating, and when the pack is removed the patient will lose heat from the surface vessels also. While the patient is resting the heart, respiratory and metabolic rates, and distribution of blood, return to normal. As long as the peripheral arterioles remain dilated and the peripheral resistance remains low, the blood pressure too will be low, but this returns to normal when the vessels constrict as the patient returns to his normal activities.

EXERCISE

The physiological effects of exercise in water are similar to those of exercise on dry land. The blood supply to the working muscles is increased, heat is evolved with each chemical change occurring during the contraction, and the muscle temperature rises. There is an increased metabolism in the muscles resulting in a greater demand for oxygen and increased production of carbon dioxide. These changes augment the similar changes brought about by the heat of the water, and both contribute towards the final effects.

The range of joint movement is either maintained or increased, and muscle power increases.

UNTOWARD EFFECTS

The physiological changes brought about by exercise in water may result in certain untoward effects of which the hydrotherapist should be aware so that she may take the necessary precautions.

A momentary rise in blood pressure occurs as the patient enters the pool; he should therefore enter slowly to minimize this effect, and the hydrotherapist should remain close to him. While the patient is in the pool his blood pressure falls and will fall still further when he rests afterwards. If the patient assumes the upright position too quickly he may feel giddy or faint. Therefore he should always get up slowly from any recumbent position either in the pool or the rest room, and the hydrotherapist should always be close to the patient as he stands up.

Chilling may occur if the patient loses heat too quickly by being exposed to a cool atmosphere before the cutaneous vessels have had time to constrict. This can be avoided by giving the patient a shower when he leaves the pool, starting with the water at pool temperature and gradually reducing it to skin temperature, and then wrapping him in a hot sheet and blanket. After the patient is dressed he should be advised to remain in room temperature for 20 minutes or so before leaving the building and, if possible, to have a drink during this time to make good the fluid loss from increased sweating.

Redistribution of blood resulting in constriction of the splanchnic vessels makes it unwise for either patient or hydrotherapist to go into the pool much less than an hour after a meal.

The patient or hydrotherapist may feel generally fatigued on leaving the pool. Although the reason for this is uncertain, the rise in temperature, possible cerebral anaemia due to the fall in blood pressure, and an accumulation of metabolites may be contributing factors. Care should be taken to build up gradually to the maximum time the patient requires in the pool. Similarly, the hydrotherapist should not remain continuously in the pool for too long—ideally, for not longer than an hour at a time.

THERAPEUTIC EFFECTS

Pool therapy is a useful method of treatment for many conditions, and has become increasingly popular during recent years. Although there are certain disadvantages, the treatment has many advantages over other forms of exercise.

Firstly, the warmth of the water in which the patient is immersed helps to relieve pain and induces relaxation. As the pain is relieved, the patient is able to move with greater comfort and the range of joint movement increases. As the warmth of the water also dilates the surface vessels and increases the blood supply to the skin, the trophic condition of the skin improves, particularly in patients with poor peripheral circulation. As the warm blood reaches the underlying muscles and their temperature rises, they contract both more easily and more strongly. Similar effects are produced by applying other forms of heat such as infra-red irradiation, but the advantage of the pool is that the heat is maintained throughout the exercise, and the muscles become fatigued less quickly.

Secondly, the buoyancy of the water supports the body and counter-balances much of the effect of gravity. This support helps to induce relaxation and to relieve pain; the feeling of weightlessness allows the patient to move his joints more freely and with less effort than if he performed the same movement on land. Combined with the effects of heat, buoyancy enables a greater range of joint movement to be achieved. A heavy patient, who is difficult to move on land, can be moved more easily and with less discomfort in the pool.

Thirdly, a finely graded progression of exercise can be obtained by using buoyancy first to assist movement, then as a support, and, finally, as a resistance. Each variation of the exercise may be modified by the use of floats, by altering the length of the weight-arm of the part being moved, by changing the speed of the movement and by creating turbulence. As a result of this fine grading a suitable exercise can be found for any strength of muscle especially those that are very weak, and can be made more difficult as muscle power increases.

The equal pressure of water on all aspects of the submerged body will support it in the upright position. This support, together with the 'weight relief' of buoyancy, will give confidence to a patient who has difficulty in walking, and indeed may enable him to walk in the pool before he can do so on land.

Swimming is a particularly useful recreational activity. The different strokes use a wide variety of muscles, and many patients who are severely handicapped out of water are surprisingly mobile in the pool. Apart from the therapeutic effect, this is of great psychological value.

Pool therapy has its disadvantages, however. Some patients are afraid of the water; there is a limit to the length of time for which both the patient and hydrotherapist can remain in the pool; it is sometimes difficult to achieve a firm fixation and so isolation of movement; a constant watch has to be kept on the chlorination of the water and the possible spread of infection; and installation and upkeep of a pool is costly. Nevertheless, the benefits of pool therapy far outweigh the disadvantages, and many patients not only gain physically from this form of treatment but also enjoy the exercise and are loath to stop even when their course of treatment is completed.

The therapeutic effects of exercise in water are, therefore: (a) to relieve pain and muscle spasm; (b) to gain relaxation; (c) to maintain or increase the range of joint movement; (d) to re-educate paralysed muscles; (e) to strengthen weak muscles and to develop their power and endurance; (f) to encourage walking and other functional and recreational activities; (g) to improve the circulation and, thus, the trophic condition of the skin, and (h) to give the patient encouragement and confidence in carrying out his exercises, thereby improving his morale.

3

Theory of Treatments

WHEN a patient arrives for his first treatment he must be examined before entering the pool and a record of all relevant information noted and subsequently kept up to date.

GENERAL PROCEDURE

After she has read the case notes the hydrotherapist takes a brief history of the onset, duration and severity of the patient's condition, notes his age and occupation and any other relevant information. The patient is asked to undress and the skin, especially of the feet, is examined for lesions such as *Tinea pedis*, open or infected wounds, or dermatitis. Minor lesions that do not constitute a contra-indication to treatment are covered with waterproof strapping. The patient is then examined specifically for the condition from which he is suffering, joint range, muscle power, coordination and balance being recorded as necessary. A more general assessment is made of his capabilities on land, this may include his ability to walk on the level or up and down stairs. Any information relevant to his disability is noted, also his build and general condition. A record is kept of all these findings for reference during treatment and for comparison at the end of the course.

The patient is then given a brief explanation of the treatment he is to receive and the reasons for it. He is also told of the approximate duration of the treatment and the length of the course. Any precautions are explained immediately before he enters the pool. As many patients are apprehensive of water care must be taken to give these patients confidence and it may be reassuring for them if they are able to watch other patients being treated before they enter the pool.

Before the patient enters the pool he is given a shower at a temperature of between 34·5° and 35·5°C (94°–96°F) which accustoms him to the temperature of the pool. He then immerses his feet in a 1 per cent chlorous solution to prevent the spread of *Tinea pedis*.

If the patient is able, he can enter the pool by walking slowly down the steps—holding the handrails on each side. If he is at all apprehensive, the hydrotherapist should walk backwards ahead of him. If he cannot manage the steps, a hoist can be used, the hydrotherapist waiting in the pool to receive him.

The length of treatment varies from 5 to 45 minutes, depending on the age and condition of the patient and the temperature of the water. Elderly patients find the temperature of the water enervating, and in combination with the physical activity, this tends to tire them, so a shorter treatment is given. Such patients usually begin with 5 to 10 minutes' treatment, increasing in length on subsequent occasions to not more than 20 or 25 minutes. Younger patients normally find that they can tolerate longer periods, up to 30 to 45 minutes. Patients suffering from conditions such as paraplegia, or an injury, will be able to stay in the pool for longer than patients suffering from systemic diseases such as rheumatoid arthritis. The length of treatment also depends on the temperature of the pool, which can vary, as desired, from 33° to 37·6°C (92°–99°F); and the lower the temperature and the younger the patient, the longer the period of immersion he can tolerate. A young paraplegic patient, for example, can withstand 45 minutes at 33°C (92°F), while an older patient with rheumatoid arthritis will tolerate only 20 minutes at 36°C (98°F).

After treatment the patient is again given a shower at 34·5° to 35·5°C, partly to cool him down and partly to wash away the chlorinated water. He is then packed in an absorbent sheet and blankets and left to rest for 20 to 30 minutes (see below). After the pack has been removed he is allowed to get up and dress slowly. Before going out he should sit for a short time in the waiting-room which is heated to about 33·3°C (65°F). A warm drink is advisable while he is resting, to replace some of the fluid lost during treatment.

A record of the date of attendance is kept for each patient, other points to note being the temperature of the water, the exercises given, the time for which the patient was in the pool and in the pack, and progressions that are made. If any untoward effect is produced this, also, must be recorded.

The pack. The pack consists of a warm absorbent sheet, a small towel and two blankets. The hydrotherapist holds the small towel in front of the patient while he removes the swimsuit. The sheet is opened lengthwise, held behind the patient and over his head; one corner is then drawn across the patient and taken over the opposite shoulder (Fig. 25 and Plates I and II). The other corner

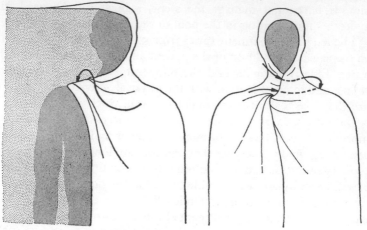

Fig. 25. Applying the pack

is taken under the first fold, tucked between this and the patient's neck, and drawn over the other shoulder. The patient then lies on a couch on top of one blanket. The small towel is pulled down, wrapped round the patient's legs, and tucked in between them. The blanket on which the patient is lying is wrapped round him, and the second one placed on top. Both blankets are loosened to prevent hyperextension of the feet. A disabled patient using sticks or crutches will not be able to stand while the sheet is being applied. In this instance a dressing-gown is held in front of him and he places one arm and then the other into each sleeve so that he is wearing it back to front. The swimsuit is then removed. The sheet, which has been placed on the couch, is then applied as above, with the patient lying down.

The pack allows the patient to cool slowly, reducing the risk of chilling. During this time the physiological changes resulting from immersion return almost to normal, and the patient can relax after the treatment in a good, functional position. The patient dries in the pack and no further drying should be necessary.

PROGRESSION OF EXERCISE

A very fine progression of exercise is possible in the pool, making use of the different effects of buoyancy, alteration in the length of the weight-arm of the moving part, and the use of floats. As on land, the rate of progression will depend on the patient's capabilities.

1. *Buoyancy assisting.* A movement is most easily performed when assisted by buoyancy and the part, such as a limb, moves from a position at right angles to the surface of the water to the horizontal position. The effect of buoyancy increases as the part approaches the horizontal, provided it is still immersed, decreasing again if the range of movement is taken beyond it. It is necessary to ensure that the patient himself performs or tries to perform the movement, otherwise the exercise becomes passive.

The progression with buoyancy assisting is made: (*a*) with a long weight-arm and (*b*) with a short weight-arm. In each instance the range and difficulty of the movement can be increased by beginning it further from the horizontal position.

2. *Buoyancy as a support.* When buoyancy is used in this way it neither assists nor resists movement of the part. At first the movement is carried out just below the surface of the water, and is then progressed by moving the part through the surface to break the surface tension. Further progression is brought about by: (*a*) having the part streamlined and moving slowly; (*b*) increasing the speed to increase turbulence; (*c*) making the part unstreamlined and slow-moving, and (*d*) by increasing the speed of movement.

3. *Buoyancy resisting.* When buoyancy is used to resist movement, the part is moved against the upthrust of the water from the horizontal position to one at right angles to the surface. If movement is continued beyond this point buoyancy will begin to assist the movement. The effect is greatest as the part moves from the horizontal, and the exercise may be progressed by beginning the movement near to the vertical position and then increasing the range to begin nearer to the horizontal.

The progression with buoyancy resisting is: (*a*) with a short weight-arm; (*b*) with a long weight-arm; (*c*) with a long weight-arm and float, moving the float from the proximal to the distal end of the part; and (*d*) by increasing the size or number of floats.

As on land, an exercise in water can be made more difficult by increasing the number of times it is performed; in addition, the hydrotherapist may give manual resistance—or assistance if required.

Strengthening the extensor muscles of the hip

1. The patient is in the prone position on a half plinth or on floats—buoyancy assisting (Figs 26, 27).

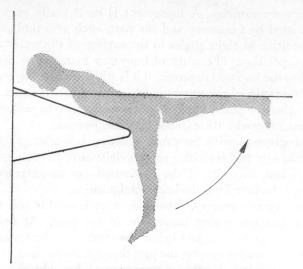

Fig. 26. Buoyancy assisting—long weight-arm

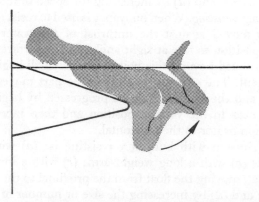

Fig. 27. Buoyancy assisting—short weight-arm

2. The patient is lying on his side on a half plinth or on floats—
buoyancy as a support (Figs 28, 29).

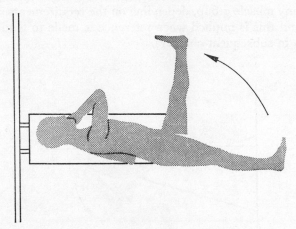

Fig. 28. Buoyancy as a support—streamlined movement

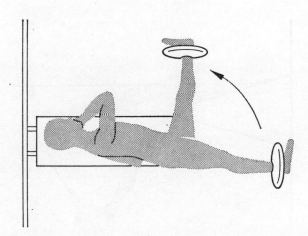

Fig. 29. Buoyancy as a support—unstreamlined movement

3. The patient lies supine on a half plinth or on floats—buoyancy resisting (Figs 30–33).

A careful record should be kept of the starting position and progression for each muscle. This progression may be adapted to almost any muscle group, depending on the requirements of treatment; and this is implied when reference is made to graded progression in subsequent chapters.

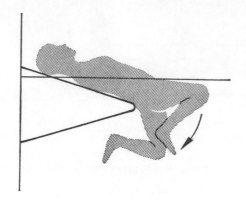

Fig. 30. Buoyancy resisting—short weight-arm

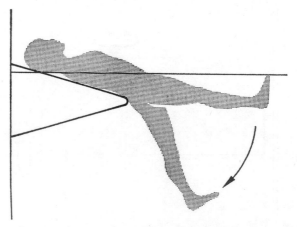

Fig. 31. Buoyancy resisting—long weight-arm

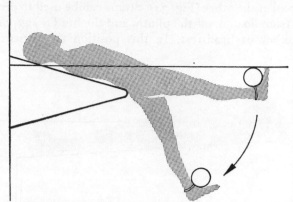

Fig. 32. Buoyancy resisting—long weight-arm and small float

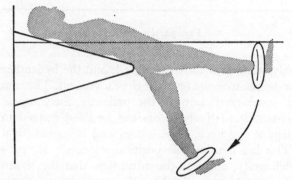

Fig. 33. Buoyancy resisting—long weight-arm and large float

STARTING POSITIONS

A variety of different starting positions is commonly used in the pool, and can be adapted to the needs of each patient. A stable starting position is sometimes difficult to achieve in water, and in such circumstances the fixation and resulting isolation of a movement is not always satisfactory. However, the use of fixed plinths, straps, or fixation by the hydrotherapist can overcome this difficulty to a great extent.

There is considerable variation in the terminology of treatment, but for ease of study the following terms are used throughout this text.

Support lying (supp: ly:). This position is adopted on a plinth or stretcher fixed to the rail of the pool at one end and to a support in the pool at the other (Fig. 34). Straps can be used to prevent the patient from floating off the plinth, and the head is supported on a small pillow or head-rest. In this position the patient is both

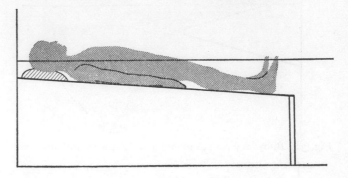

Fig. 34. Support lying

reasonably stable and fully supported, and the hydrotherapist has both hands free to assist or resist the movement. There may, however, be some restriction of the patient's knee, hip and trunk movements. Alternatively, floats can be used instead to support the patient at the neck, hips, ankles and forearms (float support lying). This is a comfortable position, especially for patients with spinal deformity, and has the advantage that the hydrotherapist can move the patient freely about the pool (Fig. 35). Nevertheless, the position is less stable than the plinth method, and fixation of the patient may be more difficult.

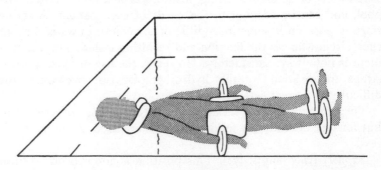

Fig. 35. Float support lying

Inclined support lying (incl: supp: ly:). In this position the patient lies on a plinth or stretcher with one end fixed to the rail of the pool, and the other lowered in the water to the required depth (Fig. 36).

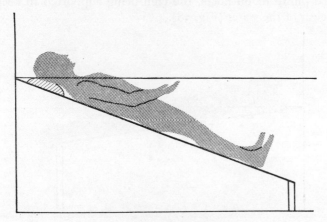

Fig. 36. Inclined support lying

Half support lying ($\frac{1}{2}$ supp: ly:). This position is taken on a half plinth with one end fixed to the rail of the pool, and the other resting against the wall under the rail. The patient's head is supported as before, and floats may be used to support one or both legs. This is comfortable for the patient, and gives him good support and firm fixation; knee and hip movements are unrestricted (Fig. 37).

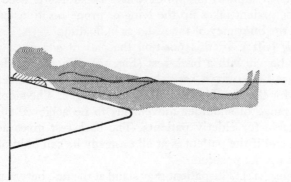

Fig. 37. Half support lying

Head support lying (h: supp: ly:). The patient's head is supported on the hydrotherapist's shoulder.

Support prone lying (supp: pr: ly:). This position is adopted on a fixed plinth or on floats, the chin being supported to keep the face clear of the water (Fig. 38).

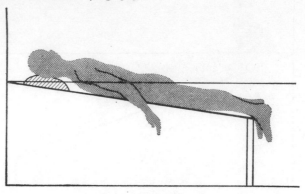

Fig. 38. Support prone lying

Half support prone lying ($\frac{1}{2}$ supp: pr: ly:). In this position the patient lies on a half stretcher, on floats or lies across a full stretcher.

Support side lying (supp: sd: ly:).

Half support side lying ($\frac{1}{2}$ supp: sd: ly:)

As in the above positions, the patient is supported on a plinth, half plinth or floats and can lie on the right or left side, e.g. support right-side lying. The advantages of these positions are similar to those of support and half support lying.

The term support is applied where apparatus is used and not when the patient takes up the lying or prone positions supported only by the buoyancy of the water as in floating.

Sitting (sitt:). In this position the patient sits on a weighted stool or bench with a back-rest (Fig. 39). When shoulder movements are being given care should be taken that the seat is low enough for the shoulder to be fully submerged. The stool enables a freer range of shoulder movements to be achieved but is less comfortable for elderly patients. The back-rest gives additional support and if the patient is at all unsteady he can hold on to it as he takes up the position.

Standing (st:). The patient may stand at the rail, between parallel bars or anywhere in the pool.

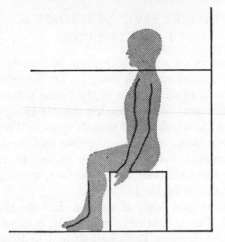

Fig. 39. Sitting

Inclined standing. The patient uses the rail of the pool to support his head and shoulders, the trunk being in an inclined plane. This position is useful for hip movements (Fig. 40).

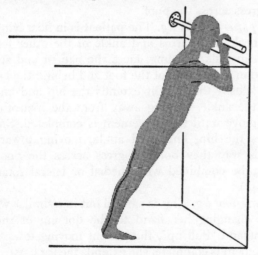

Fig. 40. Inclined standing

Kneeling. This position is adopted on a stool or on the floor of the pool if the water level is sufficiently low.

As on land derived positions from those already described may be used, by moving the arms or legs, e.g. stretch grasp support lying.

PROPRIOCEPTIVE NEUROMUSCULAR FACILITATION

Within recent years a new technique of exercise in water has been developed, based on work done by Dr Krupfer of Wildbad, Germany. This is an adaptation of the 'mass pattern' method of exercise to movement in water using muscle groups in a natural sequence rather than individual muscle groups. The principles of proprioceptive neuromuscular facilitation techniques are applied to these movements and weaker muscles can be encouraged to contract using maximal resistance, overflow, successive induction and slow reversals as on land.

With this technique floats of various sizes are the only equipment required. The hydrotherapist is in the pool with the patient and provides the fixation. Both patient and hydrotherapist move freely about the pool. The patient may move towards the hydrotherapist as, for example, in flexion patterns of the leg, or away as in extension patterns. As soon as the movement is complete the hydrotherapist moves in the same direction as the patient and so they both progress across the pool.

1. *Extension pattern of the leg.* The patient is in float lying, with a float at the neck, hips, arms and ankle of the other leg. The hydrotherapist, in walk standing, faces the patient and supports the limb in flexion on the sole of the foot and behind the knee. At the command 'Push' the patient extends the hip and knee and plantar flexes the ankle, moving away from the hydrotherapist who does not move until the movement is completed. She then passively flexes the hip, knee and ankle, moving towards the patient. In this way they both progress across the pool. The movement may be combined with medial or lateral rotation as required (Fig. 41).

2. *Flexion pattern of leg.* This is carried out in a similar way, the hydrotherapist changing her hand to the dorsum of the foot, giving the command 'Pull up', the patient moving towards her. When the movement is complete, she extends the leg passively and moves away from the patient (Fig. 42).

3. *Flexion, abduction and lateral rotation of arm.* The patient moves the arm through this pattern, moving away from the hydrotherapist who then moves up to her and the movement is repeated (Fig. 43).

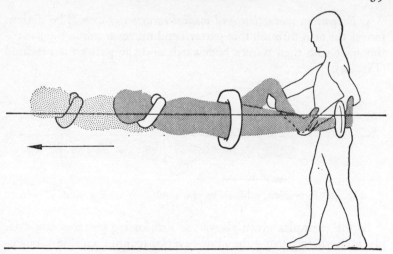

Fig. 41. Extension pattern of leg

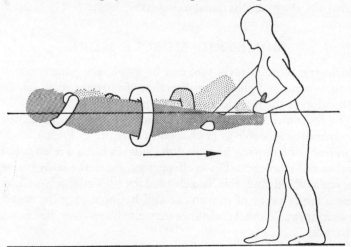

Fig. 42. Flexion pattern of leg

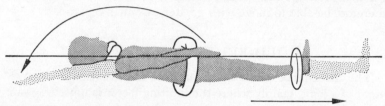

Fig. 43. Flexion, abduction and lateral rotation pattern of arm

4

4. *Extension, adduction and medial rotation of arm.* The patient moves the arm through this pattern and moves towards the hydro-therapist who then moves backwards and the pattern is repeated (Fig. 44).

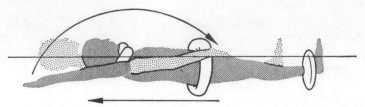

Fig. 44. Extension, adduction and medial rotation pattern of arm

In the examples given above the arm or leg patterns could be given alternately using the slow reversal technique. Trunk movements of flexion or extension combined with rotation can also be carried out, the hydrotherapist fixing at the thighs, feet or shoulders.

ISOMETRIC MUSCLE WORK

Isometric muscle work, too, can be given, the patient resisting any movement and change in direction of movement by isometric contraction of the muscle groups in turn.

The resistance to be overcome is due to the effects produced as a body moves in water as explained in Chapter 1. Pressure builds up in front of a moving body and diminishes behind it, so creating a wake and turbulence. These effects increase as the body becomes less streamlined and this is achieved by the addition of floats; using a larger range of movement and by increasing the speed of the movement. Manual resistance may also be given or, if necessary, assistance.

As with any other form of movement in the pool, the patient has the benefit of the therapeutic effects of the warm water and may therefore be able to move with greater ease than on land.

'HOLD-RELAX' TECHNIQUE

The 'hold-relax' technique is used to increase range of movement of a joint, mainly where the limiting factor is muscle spasm. It is applied in the same manner as on dry land but buoyancy may be used to assist in gaining the movement which is limited and therefore the starting position is chosen accordingly.

For example, to gain flexion of the left knee, the patient is placed in inclined prone lying on a half stretcher and the hydrotherapist stands in stride, standing on the right side of the patient, with her right foot against the patient's right heel, for stability (Fig. 45).

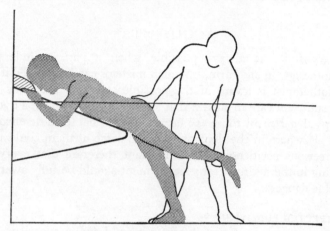

Fig. 45. To gain flexion of knee

The hydrotherapist's right hand steadies the left side of the pelvis and her left hand is placed on the anterior aspect of the lower leg. The knee is bent as far as possible in the pain free range, either actively or passively. At the command 'hold', the hydrotherapist applies resistance with the left hand and the knee extensor muscles contract strongly isometrically. At the command 'relax', she releases the resistance and steadies the lower leg as the extensor muscles relax and buoyancy assists further flexion of the knee. The patient may reinforce this by bending the knee actively, and at the same time proprioceptive stimulation may be added by applying resistance to the posterior aspect of the lower leg.

Although it is preferable to have buoyancy assisting the movement into the limited range this technique may be given with buoyancy neutralized. As on dry land the movement into the limited range may be gained passively; by a free active movement or a resisted movement.

4
Dangers and Precautions

ACCIDENTS

AN ACCIDENT is always possible when a patient undergoes physiotherapy in any form, but such mishaps can be avoided if the physiotherapist is aware of the possible causes of accidents and takes sufficient care to ensure that they do not happen. In a hydrotherapy department there are hazards additional to those encountered elsewhere in the department, and some of them could produce serious accidents. It is important therefore that everyone working in the hydrotherapy department should be fully aware of possible dangers.

UNEXPECTED SUBMERSION

Unexpected submersion in water is an alarming experience for anyone and should this occur when a patient is receiving hydrotherapy it could destroy completely his confidence in this form of treatment, particularly if he is at all apprehensive of water. There are several ways in which it could occur; either while actually in the pool or on entering or leaving it. While in the pool, the patient could slip and overbalance although this danger is reduced in modern pools by the use of non-slip tiles. The patient might be knocked over by another patient or hydrotherapist. This is most likely to happen if the pool is overcrowded or if a patient is allowed to swim across the pool on his back without making sure that there is a clear space in the water. Care therefore should be taken that the pool does not become overcrowded and—although the number of patients that can be treated at one time will vary with the size of the pool—sufficient space should be available to allow patients and staff to move about freely. Swimming should only be allowed when there is sufficient space available.

When walking on crutches in a pool the danger of overbalancing is greater than on land as the legs tend to float to the surface owing to the effect of buoyancy. Patients walking on crutches should be carefully instructed to take only small steps, both with the feet and crutches.

The effect of buoyancy also allows the patient's legs to float to the surface if he sits down too quickly or too far from the seat. Patients must therefore be warned to stand right back against the stool, to bend their knees and hips, and then to sit down slowly. If a back-rest is available the patient can use it to steady himself.

If a stretcher is used it must be fixed securely at each end to prevent it from sinking under the patient's weight. Both ends should be checked before a patient gets on to the stretcher.

A handrail round the pool provides the patient with a means of support but the hydrotherapist should be in the pool nearby, ready to give help and support to the patient if necessary.

In a pool of graded depth it is possible for a patient to walk un-expectedly into deeper water, and for a child to walk beyond his depth. This is more likely in a pool that is graded in steps rather than sloped towards the deep end, but in each instance patients should be warned if the pool is graded. In the former type of pool patients are less likely to mistake the depth of water if different coloured tiles are used to mark the edges of each step.

If the patient enters the pool by hoist care must be taken to ensure that he does not fall off it—the chair or stretcher must clear the edge of the pool before being lowered, and the patient's legs must also clear the rim of the pool. If the more rigid type of chair is used, the bar across the front should be securely fastened; however, with the more modern, sling-type chair, the patient is less likely to fall as the material of the chair 'moulds' itself to some extent around the patient, so providing extra support. The hydro-therapist should be in the pool to receive the patient, as this not only gives him greater confidence but also minimizes the danger of falling as the patient leaves the chair for the water.

When the patient enters the pool by the steps he may lose his footing as he moves from the last step into the pool. The refraction of the water makes it difficult to appreciate when the lowest step is reached, so, as in the graded pool, the last step should be marked clearly in a different colour; better still, tiles of different colour should be used for all the steps. A handrail on each side of the steps will give the patient support as he enters the pool.

FALLS

Although a patient might fall in any part of a hospital building, the likelihood is greater in the hydrotherapy department, as the floor may be wet and slippery. Falls are most liable to occur on the surrounds of the pool, in the rest room and in the shower cubicle. The patient could also fall over accessory apparatus, such as a float if it is left lying on the floor. To prevent accidents, the tiles on the area around the pool and in the shower are usually ridged or studded, and unlikely to become slippery. In the shower cubicle, a rail fixed to the wall, approximately three feet from the ground, will minimize the danger of falls. Other floor covering, such as linoleum, is often used in the rest room, and should it become wet it should be dried at once; otherwise it could become dangerously slippery. If linoleum and similar types of floor covering require polish to preserve them, a non-slip polish should be used.

BURNS AND SCALDS

These are infrequent accidents, but they may occur if hot water pipes are exposed or if a thermostat fails to regulate the temperature of the water in a shower. As a precaution, therefore, all exposed water pipes within the patients' or hydrotherapists' reach should be lagged, and thermostats should be checked and overhauled regularly.

PROCEDURE SHOULD AN ACCIDENT OCCUR

Should an accident occur the appropriate measures should be taken without delay.

If a patient becomes submerged in the pool he must be helped immediately, his head being kept above water and supported by the hydrotherapist. He is taken out of the pool, using a stretcher and hoist if necessary. He should rest on a couch and be wrapped in warm sheets as some degree of shock is likely. If he is badly shocked, distressed, or has injured himself in any way, a doctor must be called to examine him. If he is not badly shocked he may be allowed to rest quietly for half an hour or so, given a hot drink and allowed to go home. All patients who have had an accident of any kind will require help and reassurance from the hydrotherapist, but patients who have been inadvertently submerged are naturally frightened by their experience and most will require much encouragement from the hydrotherapist before receiving further treatment.

It is also possible, although unlikely, for a patient to drown. In any case in which a patient has been submerged for any length of time, artificial respiration may be required immediately, and a second person should call a doctor. As a precaution in case of accident, there should never be less than two hydrotherapists in the department when there is a patient in the pool, and all staff working in the department must be proficient in at least one method of artificial respiration.

Should a patient fall, he must be seen by a doctor before leaving the building. First aid may be given by the hydrotherapy staff but the doctor is responsible for subsequent treatment, and must therefore be consulted.

A complete record of all accidents must be made, including treatment given and the names and addresses of any witnesses. These records must be kept for 3 years after the accident occurs, as this is the statutory period during which a patient may institute legal proceedings against the staff and hospital.

INFECTIONS

All infectious or contagious disease can spread from one person to another in a hydrotherapy department, as elsewhere, and the precautions customary in hospitals must be taken by the hydrotherapist.

All contagious and infectious skin diseases are a contra-indication (see Chapter 6) to pool treatment and patients with such conditions must not be given pool therapy until the skin condition has been cured. If there is any sign of possible infection in either staff or patient, the physician in charge of the department should be consulted before that person is allowed in the pool.

To minimize the spread of infection, the pool is chlorinated regularly, either by a chlorifier incorporated into the circulating mechanism or by adding chlorous manually. In addition, a regular bacteriological analysis of the water is carried out. All swimsuits must be washed each time they are used, and all bathing shoes and caps sterilized. Similarly, dressing-gowns, sheets and towels can be used once only before washing. Blankets do not come into

contact with the patients but should be changed daily; the cotton
cellular type is washed very easily.

There are two conditions which are particularly likely to flourish
in the hydrotherapy department and special precautions must be
taken against *Tinea pedis* and ringworm.

TINEA PEDIS

Tinea pedis is a water-borne fungus infection and may spread
very rapidly in such places as swimming-pools and hydrotherapy
departments. There are two types, the vesicular and the inter-
triginous. The vesicular type grows on the corneal layer of the skin
but may produce changes in the underlying epidermis, causing
vesicle formation. This type of infection frequently begins under
the arch of the foot and spreads to the heel and even the dorsum
of the foot. It is characterized by an erythema under which the
vesicles can be seen, first as small white spots but later as purulent
vesicles. The infection may be unilateral or bilateral. The inter-
triginous type begins between the toes, usually the fourth and fifth,
and may spread to the other toes and adjacent parts of the sole of
the foot. The skin appears white and soft and then peels off, leaving
a reddened area beneath.

As the condition is highly contagious every care should be taken
to prevent its spread. All patients' feet should be examined at their
first attendance and signs of infection should be reported to the
doctor in charge of the patient before treatment is given. The
physician in charge of the hydrotherapy department must also be
informed immediately of any suspected case of *Tinea pedis*.
Neither patients nor staff should be allowed to walk anywhere in
the department without shoes. These should be worn once only,
and then sterilized in a chlorous solution before being used again.
A foot-bath containing chlorous solution should be kept at the top
of the steps leading into the pool, and everyone should immerse
their feet before going into the pool.

TINEA CAPITIS

Tinea capitis (ringworm) is now relatively rare in the United
Kingdom, but infections do occur and can spread rapidly if proper
precautions are not taken. Swimming caps used by patients and
staff must be sterilized immediately after use in a chlorous or
other disinfectant solution. However, most staff, and many

patients, prefer to use their own bathing caps, and these need not be sterilized.

The disinfectant used for sterilizing caps and shoes will vary from one hospital to another. One method is to use a chlorine solution such as Voxan, 20 ml of which is mixed with 5 l. of water.

5
Pools, Tanks and Accessory Equipment

THE hydrotherapy department is a self-contained unit, with its own changing, rest and utility rooms, and ample storage space for linen and equipment. The department should be designed with as few doors as possible, and these, and the corridors, should be wide enough to allow easy transit of stretchers and wheelchairs. There should also be sufficient room to turn stretchers round if necessary, and a place for the temporary parking of stretchers and wheelchairs. The size of the department depends on the demands of each hospital, and the type of patient undergoing treatment.

The pool area should be well lighted, preferably by natural light, and designed to give a feeling of spaciousness. The pool itself should be large enough to allow the patient to progress throughout his full rehabilitation programme, from using the full support of a stretcher to partial support, then on to walking and, ideally, to swimming and other recreational activities. A pool 8 by 10 ft can accommodate, at most, two patients and a hydrotherapist at one time, but its use is limited compared with a pool of 12 by 20 ft which can take seven or eight patients and three hydrotherapists. Thus the larger the pool the greater the use to which it can be put. When swimming is an integral part of the patient's rehabilitation, as in the treatment of spinal injuries, a much larger area of, say, 30 by 15 ft is necessary. According to a survey conducted by K. R. Greenlees* on therapy pools in Britain, their sizes vary from 80 sq ft to 350 sq ft, the largest group (32 per cent) having an area of 150 to 200 sq ft.

The pool area is usually kept at 23·9°C (75°F), and the changing

* Available from Arthur F. Houghton & Associates, 14 St Andrews Road, West Town, Blackwell, nr. Bristol.

and rest rooms at 18·3°C (65°F). Ventilation should prevent too much condensation, and to this end, the ceiling and walls have a special surface. Humidity is kept at 50 to 60 per cent.

POOLS AND TANKS

At present, pools are built with a reinforced concrete shell, a layer of asphalt and a second layer of reinforced concrete. Tiles, mosaic, fibreglass or plastic are used as lining materials; if tiles are used they have a rough finish, or the surface is ridged or studded to ensure that they are slip proof.

Prefabricated fibreglass pools are now available in standard sizes, and these can be enlarged by adding another section. This type of pool may well become cheaper and easier to install in the future.

SUNKEN AND RAISED POOLS

Pools can be either sunk or raised, the former type being constructed at promenade level while the latter is surmounted by a 2 ft 8 in wall (approximately waist height). The choice is largely a matter of individual preference, but a good case can be made for each type. In a new building there is little difference in the cost of erection, but a raised pool may be a more suitable choice for installation in an existing building. Some engineers believe that the raised pool is easier to maintain and keep clean.

The sunken pool (Plate III) is surmounted by a kerb 8 or 9 in high, and has steps by which the patient can enter. These may be built into the pool or made of teak and fixed to one wall. In this type of pool the patient has fewer steps to negotiate than in the raised pool, and since the water level is lower relative to the height of the ceiling, air is able to circulate more freely, and the effect is less claustrophobic. Use of a sunken pool makes it necessary for the hydrotherapist to be in the pool while treating the patient. Many authorities believe this ensures the best possible treatment; fixation of the patient by the hydrotherapist is firmer, and she has more control over his movements.

The raised or free-standing pool (Plate IV) has an outer wall 8 in wide and 2 ft 8 in high. It slopes slightly outward towards the foot to a recess at floor level under which the therapist can tuck her feet when she leans over the wall to a patient in the pool (Fig. 46).

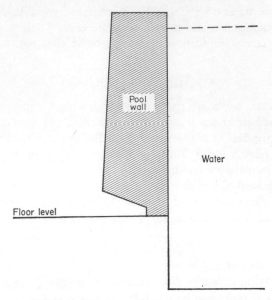

Fig. 46. Cross-section of a raised pool

With this type of pool, communication with the patient is easier, and in a busy department with a small staff, it may also be an advantage to control some patients from outside the pool thus allowing the hydrotherapist to treat more patients than with a sunken pool where her time in the pool itself must be restricted. On the other hand, fixation, and thus control, of the patient is less localized from the side.

Pool floor and depth. The floor of the pool may be level, sloping or graded in two or three depths. A level floor allows freedom of range over the whole pool, and a four-foot depth of water gives sufficient buoyancy for all patients. In addition, this type of floor allows most adult patients to walk with confidence, and enables even the shortest therapist to maintain a firm foothold and therefore a good control of the patient during exercise. In some pools the depth of the water can be altered, though it may take time for the water to reach the correct temperature at the new level.

A minimum *depth* of 4 ft 6 in is required for the treatment of paraplegics to avoid flail limbs touching the bottom. For children the ideal depth varies from 2 ft 9 in to 4 ft. The shallower end of the range is advisable if the children are to walk in the pool, though some hydrotherapists prefer to have the advantage of the increased buoyancy of deeper water.

The usual *gradient* for a pool with a sloping floor is 1 in 15. A sloping floor can be most satisfactory in a large pool, and where swimming plays an important part both in rehabilitation and recreational activities; all patients will benefit from performing their exercises in the depth of water most suitable to their height.

A *graded floor* usually has three depths of water, stepped lanes running the length of the pool at the 2 ft 9 in, 3 ft 3 in and at 4 ft marks. The demarcation between each step must be made very clearly visible by using tiles of different colours on the edge of each step. The graded pool is particularly useful if both adults and children are being treated. The grading is also an asset in progressing exercises for walking from deep to shallower water, with a resulting increase in weight bearing. In this type of pool, however, only a limited area of the water is sufficiently deep to give the effect of maximum buoyancy.

Use of a bay is an alternative method of varying the depth of a pool, a free-standing rectangular pool being extended to give one, or more, shallow bays, each to accommodate one patient for exercise. The bays are usually 6 to 8 ft wide and 18 in to 2 ft 9 in deep. They may be used as an introduction to pool therapy in cases where the hydrostatic pressure of deeper water could cause respiratory distress, or to give the therapist good control of a very nervous patient.

TANKS

A Hubbard tank (Plate V) is often installed where space is limited, and it may also be used as an addition to an existing pool. The tank is usually 8 ft 6 in long, trefoil- or keyhole-shaped, and 7 ft across at its widest point. The waist of the tank is 2 ft 8 in and the depth of water varies from 2 ft to 2 ft 6 in. The wings allow for arm movements. The patient can be treated on the stretcher on which he is lifted into the tank, and, as the rim of the tank is waist high it is easy for the therapist to handle the patient. The water can be changed after each patient, as is necessary in the treatment of burns or septic conditions.

To provide local treatment for stiff joints and muscular spasm, an underwater jet can be installed. This operates at a temperature 6°C (10°F) above that of the pool and at a pressure of 10 lb per square inch. It is unfortunately less easily fitted to pools controlled by continuous heating and filtration plants, but could be a useful adjunct to a small pool.

HANDRAILS

Whatever the type of pool, it is surrounded by a handrail made of stainless steel, plastic coated metal or of teak approximately $1\frac{1}{2}$ in in diameter and fixed 2 to 3 in from the pool wall, at water level. If the water level is to be varied an additional rail is desirable at the alternative water level.

STEPS

The steps leading to the pool have 6-in risers and there should be a handrail on each side. The width of the steps should be narrow enough for the patient to hold both handrails when entering and leaving the pool. If the pool is of the raised type, a second flight of steps is necessary to enable the ambulant patient to reach the top of the surrounding wall.

FOOT-BATH

Everyone entering the pool has to immerse his feet in a solution of chlorinated water, and this is provided by a foot-bath placed near to the steps (Fig. 47); it is best built into the floor with its own taps and drainage.

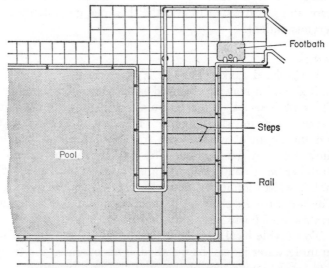

Fig. 47. Steps and foot-bath from above

SIDEWALKS

The sidewalks surrounding the pool are at least 4 ft wide on three sides, and 8 ft or more on the fourth side where the hoist and steps are placed, and there is room for stretchers and chairs. Slip-proof, ridged or studded tiles are used for the flooring, which is very slightly sloped to allow effective drainage of surplus water.

WATER TEMPERATURE AND PURIFICATION

The temperature at which the pool is kept is influenced by the general atmospheric conditions and the ventilation of the department as a whole. Humidity increases as the water temperature rises, and this can prove fatiguing for patients and staff. Pool temperatures vary from 34° to 37°C (94°-98°F), according to the specific need. For cases of orthopaedic and spinal injury, the pool is usually between 34° and 36°C (94-96°F), whereas arthritic conditions are treated more satisfactorily at a temperature of 36°-37°C (96°-98°F). Thermometers and hygrometers should be available in the department so that water temperature and humidity can be tested.

If the pool is very small it is emptied and refilled immediately for re-use. With a large pool, however, a plant is required for heating, filtering, sterilizing and exchanging the water, the plant being designed to give a complete water turnover every four hours or less.*

From the pool outlet the water passes through a coarse strainer before being pumped into the filter, and circulated through the calorifier, which heats the water to the desired temperature; finally, the sterilizing agent is added. The water is aerated by passing it through a closed chamber into which air is blown—this helps to maintain bacterial purity and gives a sparkle to the water.

The chlorination of the water should give a result of 0·5 to 0·75 parts per million of free chlorine, too high a concentration acting as an irritant to the skin. Alum and the chlorine used for sterilization and coagulation are acid forming, and as water purified by continuous filtration should be kept slightly alkaline with a pH value of 7·2-8·0 it is necessary to add an alkali such as soda ash or lime to the water before it reaches the sand filter.

The residual chlorine content and pH value are tested two or

* *See* 'Purification of Swimming Baths', H.M.S.O.

three times throughout the day, and, in addition, a bacteriological analysis of the water is made at regular intervals. The plant attendant should keep a daily log recording the hours for which the plant is working, the number of people using the pool, and the results of the checks on the chlorine content and pH of the water. From this record can be calculated the amount of chlorine and alkalis to be added to the water to maintain its purification.

If the pool is without sterilizing plant, the chlorine is added directly at regular intervals during the day. The hydrotherapist can check the residual chlorine by using a simple apparatus based upon the orthotolodine test.*

ACCESSORY EQUIPMENT

The pool itself has a minimum of fixed apparatus, and a variety of accessory equipment is therefore necessary.

For sunken pools, a hoist or gantry with overhead rails is used to lift handicapped patients in and out of the water (Plate VI). Electrically or pneumatically powered units are now superseding the mechanically controlled types. With raised pools and tanks a hydraulic lift is more usual. The lifting device is so designed that it can be worked by one operator, who can, at the same time, control the patient in the chair or stretcher.

Although stretchers may be required for some patients, it is more usual to lift the patient in a specially designed chair or nylon sling which maintains him in a sitting posture. Many patients prefer this, and feel more confident during the lift if they are in a sitting position. The use of wheelchairs rather than stretchers also saves space, and is thus helpful in a busy department. When the patient can only lie on a stretcher, this can also be attached to the hoist.

Stretchers or plinths for use in the pool are best made of tubular steel with a nylon mesh cover and can be hooked on to the rail of the pool. A full-length stretcher can be supported on a platform at the far end, the near end being hooked over the pool rail; a half-length stretcher supports itself against the pool wall; in each case the angle of the stretcher can be adjusted.

* Orthotolodine test. A small measured sample of pool water is added to a measured sample of chemical reagent. After shaking well, compare with colour chart provided.

PLATES

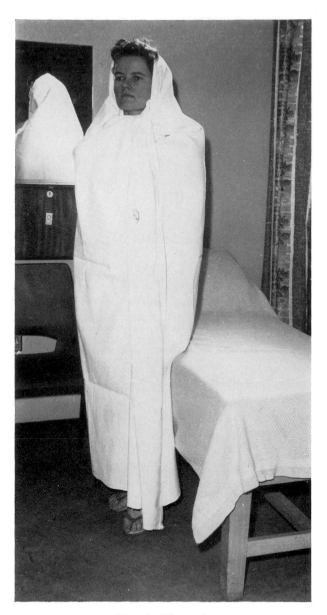

Plate I. The pack

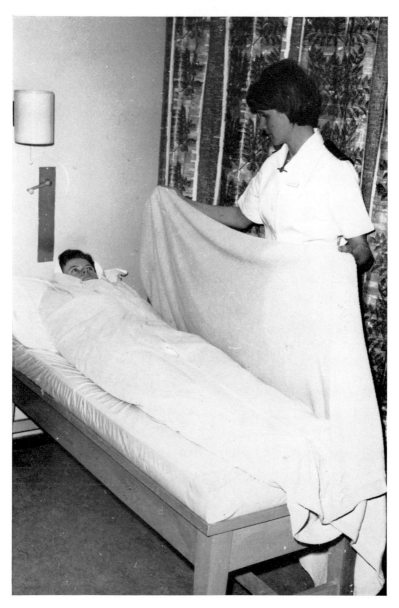

Plate II. The pack

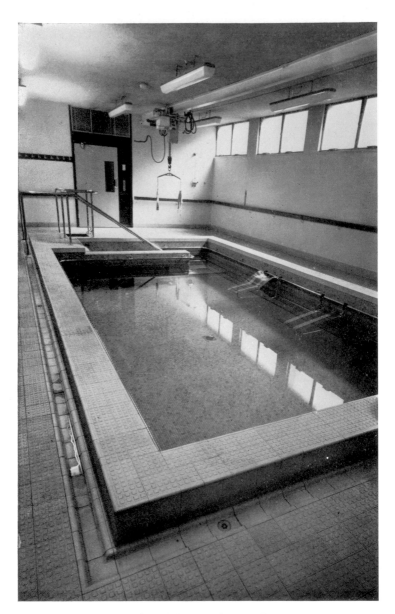

Plate III. A sunken pool

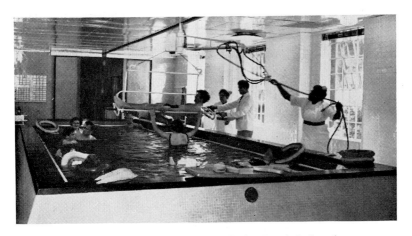

Plate IV. The pool at St Benedict's Hospital, London

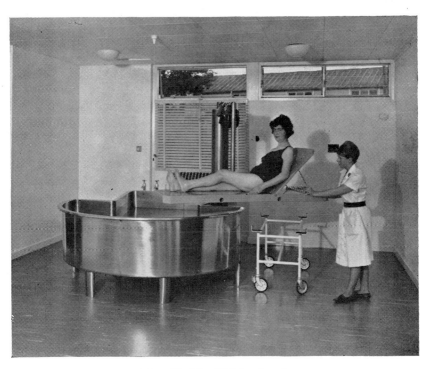

Plate V. The Hubbard tank

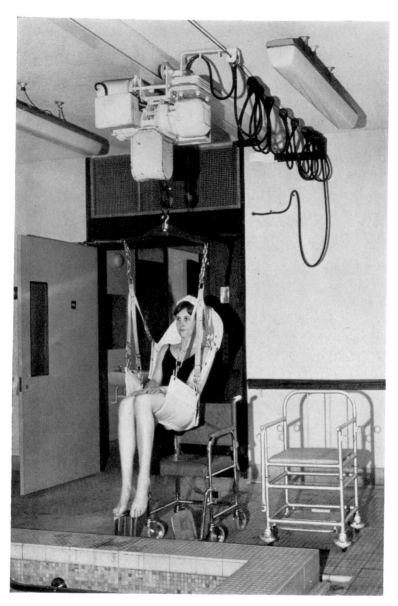

Plate VI. An electrically operated hoist

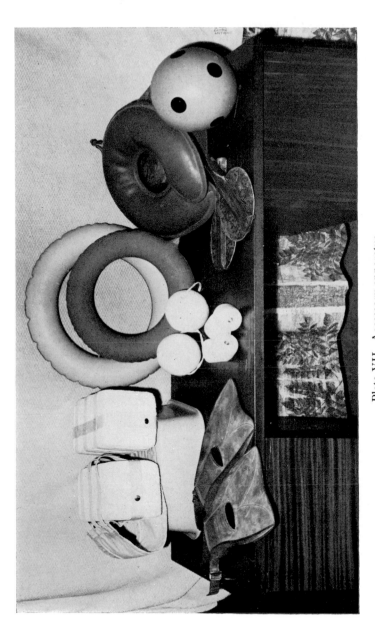

Plate VII. Accessory apparatus

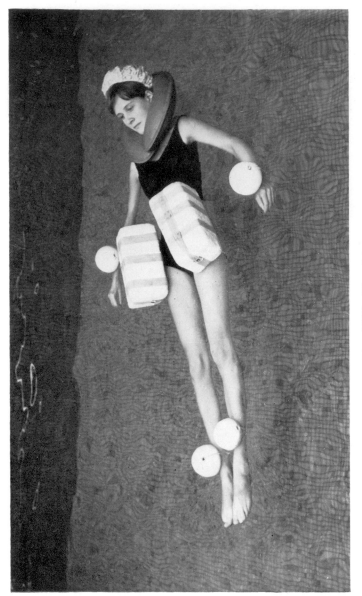

Plate VIII. Float lying

Parallel bars are useful and to avoid taking unnecessary space in the pool a second rail may be hooked across the pool parallel to the handrail whenever bars are needed.

Teak is used to make stools and benches which are weighted to keep them on the floor of the pool. They should be of varying height to allow the shoulders of patients to be immersed fully.

Head-rests attached to the rail are very useful but an entirely satisfactory design has proved difficult to achieve. An inflated semicircular ring is used to support the head of a patient floating on his back, and should be sufficiently buoyant to prevent the hair from becoming wet.

Floats are available in a variety of materials. Cork, or various plastic materials such as Jablite or polystyrene may be used in different sizes in combination with canvas slings or cords. Block floats, 12 in by 4 in square and attached to each end of a canvas sling, may be used to support the trunk, while balls of varying diameter attached to cords, are used for the limbs (Plates VII and VIII).

Rubber rings are available in diameters ranging from 12 in to 24 in, and can be used for both trunk and limbs. During arm exercises, 'ping-pong' bats of light wood or metal, and of varying sizes (5 in, 7 in, 9 in) are used to give a streamlined or unstreamlined effect. 'Flippers' can be used, similarly, on the feet.

Patients often have to be fixed to stretchers or stools by webbing straps. These are usually 3 in wide and 4 to 5 ft long; they may have Velcro fastenings at each end or a buckle at one end.

Crutches and sticks are made of metal or wood weighted at the foot.

Although some patients may prefer to use their own swimsuits or trunks, it is more practical to provide them. Ideally, these should be of the type that is removed easily, allows unrestricted movement and enables the hydrotherapist to see the joints moving. A 'bikini' style with Velcro fastenings fulfils all these requirements and, if made of stretch material in small, medium and large sizes, will fit most patients. This type of swimsuit has the additional advantage of being easy to wash and dry. A regulation swimsuit in stretch material is most suitable for staff.

Light cotton dressing-gowns must be provided for patients, and thicker, towelling gowns or track suits are needed by the staff.

Shoes need to be washable and easy to put on and remove.

6

Mules with rope soles and spacious canvas tops are suitable for patients with severe foot deformities. For other patients and for staff, the best type to use is one with a rubber sole held in position by a strap passing over the forefoot, and secured between the first and second toes (Fig. 48).

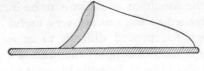

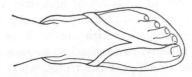

Fig. 48. Two suitable sandals for pool use

A large stock of sheets, towels and blankets is required. Absorbent twill sheets or turkish towels 60 in by 80 in and turkish or huckaback towels 32 in by 18 in are required. Blankets must be easy to wash; cotton cellular weaves are ideal. If orderlies are attached to the department they will help patients to dress and undress, wash and dry swimsuits, sterilize shoes and caps, and be responsible for the linen. The hydrotherapist can then give her undivided attention to the treatment of her patients.

Patients and staff must take a shower on entering and leaving the pool. The showers should therefore be near the pool, and those for the patients' use are most conveniently sited near the pool steps and hoist. The shower, which is thermostatically controlled, is fixed to the wall at a height of about 5 ft, and the spray head should be angled so that patients can shower without getting their hair wet. A flexible tube and spray should be available for the use of stretcher and chair patients. Handrails are fixed round the walls for security. The floor, which is made of non-slip material, slopes sufficiently to allow the water to drain away.

ADDITIONAL ACCOMMODATION

In the rest room each cubicle is furnished with a well-padded couch approximately 20 in high, and a mattress covered with waterproof material. A locker and key is provided in which the patient may hang up his clothes and leave any valuables while he is in the pool. Ideally the number of rest cubicles should exceed the maximum number of patients that the pool can accommodate.

A large well-heated linen room, fitted with slatted shelves, is also necessary as a large quantity of linen is used in a hydrotherapy department. The temperature in the linen room must be high enough to warm the sheets and towels used for packing the patient and for airing the swimsuits, slippers and dressing-gowns used in the department.

The quantity of linen required will vary with local conditions, depending on the number of staff and patients involved and the laundry facilities available. However, a large sheet, small towel, swimsuit, dressing-gown and slippers are required by each patient and a large towel, swimsuit, dressing-gown or track suit and slippers for each member of the staff. Two blankets are needed for each couch, together with two or more pillows and pillow cases.

The necessary store cupboards for accessory equipment should, preferably, be close to the pool. They can be housed in the utility room with a sink unit, washing machine and spin dryer, which can be used to wash and dry swimsuits, shoes and caps, for both patients and staff.

Lavatories and washbasins are needed for the patients: the door of one lavatory must be wide enough to take a wheelchair, and one should have a raised seat, and handrails on the adjacent walls.

A separate staff changing-room is needed, equipped with shower, lavatory and washbasin, and a locker for each member of the staff.

The hydrotherapist in charge is responsible for the treatment of patients, for her staff both trained and untrained, for the equipment that is used, for the smooth running of the department, and for the appointments and treatments records. She should do her best to encourage understanding and consideration between staff and patients for the harmonious working of her department depends greatly upon the successful cooperation between all members of the unit.

6

Indications and Contra-indications

INDICATIONS

IN RECENT years pool therapy has become much more widely used in the treatment of diseases affecting the locomotor system. Its value is due chiefly to three factors. The water is comfortably warm and as a result pain is reduced and patients can move with greater comfort. The water is buoyant and therefore will support the body, producing a partial weightlessness, again enabling a patient to move more easily than on land. This buoyancy also allows for a very finely graded progression of activity.

Pool therapy is therefore a method of treatment that is of considerable benefit to those patients whose signs and symptoms fall in certain categories. It will be indicated for patients suffering from rheumatic disorders such as osteo- and rheumatoid arthritis, with stiff and painful joints and often with difficulty in walking. Patients with neurological disorders such as hemiplegia, paraplegia and polyneuritis resulting in spasticity or flaccidity of muscle will also benefit from a course of pool treatment. Following orthopaedic surgery and injury such as a fracture, particularly of the back and lower limbs, exercise in water will do much to restore joint mobility and muscle power and to help the patient to return to normal activity.

The deep pool too has a recreational value, and here it is of particular value in the treatment of children. They are often more ambulant in water than out of it and a child unable to walk may be taught to swim. One of the objects of treating a child suffering, for example, from cerebral palsy is to make him fearless in water and therefore able to enjoy this form of recreation.

Patients may become too dependent on this form of treatment so that it is usually advisable to limit the length of a course to a specific number of treatments. In many instances too, it may be given in conjunction with exercises on land or it may be advisable to alternate pool therapy with other forms of physiotherapy.

CONTRA-INDICATIONS

There are few absolute contra-indications to this type of treatment.

GENERAL CONSIDERATION

It will be obvious that severely debilitated patients, or those with an active febrile condition will be unsuitable for pool therapy, as will those who are incontinent of faeces. Incontinence of urine is not normally considered to be a contra-indication but it might be advisable to increase the chlorination of the water if the incontinence is considerable. Epileptic patients, while not being completely excluded, should be chosen with care and constantly supervised while in the water. Although there is no physiological reason why a patient or hydrotherapist should not go into the pool while menstruating it may be impracticable for some women during the first day.

DERMATOLOGICAL CONDITIONS

Patients with a contagious skin infection should be excluded from treatment because of the risk to others, particularly those with *Tinea pedis* (see Chapter 4) which is a waterborne infection. The same remarks apply to those with infected wounds or discharging sinuses. Indolent ulcers, if small, may be covered and sealed by a sticky waterproof dressing if it is important that pool exercises should be given.

A few patients develop skin eruptions due to sensitivity to the presence of chlorination in the pool, and such patients are generally unsuitable for such treatment.

CARDIOVASCULAR DISORDERS

Owing to the resistance of the water, treatment in the deep pool demands a fair degree of exercise tolerance, and those with incipient or established cardiac failure from any cause should be excluded, as should those with severe peripheral arterial disease.

Whereas patients who have had a cerebral thrombosis may normally be treated easily without risk, those who have suffered a cerebral haemorrhage should not be given this type of treatment for at least 3 weeks after evidence of bleeding has ceased.

Moderate hypertension is not a contra-indication, but some hypertension involves the same risk for such patients as any other form of exercise. Patients with hypotension should be treated with caution since a further fall of blood pressure may occur during treatment.

RESPIRATORY DISEASE

Patients with respiratory disease will be limited to those whose exercise tolerance is sufficient for them to receive treatment without distress—in general, those with a vital capacity of more than 1500 cm³. Those with active lung infection such as tuberculosis are unsuitable for treatment.

As will be seen from the above, not only should the probable benefit of pool therapy be assessed for each patient, but a careful assessment of the general medical condition should be made before such treatment is prescribed.

7
The Treatment of
Rheumatic Disorders

THE signs and symptoms common to most rheumatic conditions
are pain, limitation of movement, muscle weakness, deformity and
a decrease in functional ability. Hydrotherapy is of great value in
the treatment of many of these conditions, for the warmth of the
water will decrease both pain and muscle spasm, while its buoyancy allows non-weight exercises to be given, so relieving strain on
the joints.

SIGNS AND SYMPTOMS

Pain in and around the affected joints leads to tension and
spasm in certain muscle groups acting on them. In the pool, pain
is relieved by the warmth of the water surrounding the joint, this
helps relaxation so bringing further relief of pain. The buoyancy
provided by the water supports the part and so decreases the strain
on the affected weight-bearing joints.

Limitation of movement and stiffness in the joints is decreased,
partly by the relief of pain and muscle spasm, and partly by the
support of buoyancy during movement.

Muscle weakness. The muscle groups surrounding the affected
part can be strengthened by graduated exercises in the pool. At
first buoyancy is used to assist the muscle, but gradually the effect
of buoyancy is diminished until the exercise can be performed
using buoyancy as a resistance.

Deformity is a characteristic of certain conditions. Again, the
warmth of the water helps the muscles to relax and as a result,
further corrections of the deformity can be achieved. In addition,
owing to the buoyancy of the water the affected muscles do not
have to contend with the pull of gravity.

Decrease in functional ability. The support of the water helps to restore muscle function by making movement easier, thus building up the patient's confidence in his ability to perform similar movements on land.

OSTEO-ARTHRITIS

This condition usually affects the weight-bearing joints in the body, mainly the hip and knee. Some or all of the above signs and symptoms will be present in most patients. In more advanced stages of the disease the deformity will be flexion, adduction and lateral rotation of the hip and flexion of the knee and, therefore, apparent shortening of the leg. The strength of muscles around the affected joints can be built up by graduated exercise making use of buoyancy and using floats in the later stages of treatment. Range can be maintained and increased using the freedom of movement offered by the water with the support given to the limbs by buoyancy.

Back exercises should be included in the treatment as a compensatory scoliosis or lordosis is one complication of an osteo-arthritic hip. In addition, a strong and mobile lumbar spine is desirable to take the extra strain imposed when the hip is stiff and painful. In later stages of treatment the patient can be taught swimming movements for the legs, and, eventually, to swim across the pool.

Functional difficulties of osteo-arthritic patients are generally concerned with walking and climbing stairs, and much can be done to re-educate such patients in the pool. Many patients are more mobile in water than on land and this gives them greater confidence and a sense of achievement. This encourages them to try the same movements on land.

The patient can use the steps of the pool to strengthen the muscles used in going up and down stairs. The steps become increasingly difficult to climb as patients leave the pool and have to support more and more of their body weight. Conversely, the descent becomes easier as more of the body is covered by water.

If the condition does not respond to conservative treatment, an operation may become necessary. Pool therapy is a useful pre-operative treatment to build up the strength of muscles acting on the affected joint, and to increase its range of movement.

SUGGESTED TREATMENT FOR THE KNEES

EARLY STAGE

During this stage the emphasis is mainly on strengthening the quadriceps and increasing the range of movement in the knee joint—using buoyancy to assist and, later, to resist the movement. Treatment usually begins with the patient supported on a half-plinth. This position keeps the lower limbs free of support and unrestricted in their movement, while giving the patient the re-assurance of having the upper half of his body supported before progressing to a less fixed starting position. Exercises such as these may be given:

1. Half support lying—quadriceps contractions.
2. Half support lying—knee bending and stretching.
3. Half support lying—leg parting and closing.
4. Half support side lying—bending and stretching upper-most knee. Repeat on other side.
5. Reach grasp standing—alternate knee raising and lower-ing.
6. Stride standing—rhythmic stabilization progressing to walk standing and standing.
7. Walk with support of hydrotherapist or parallel bars.

The patient can also be taught, and encouraged to practise correction posture. If parallel bars are available, walking can be begun between them and then progressed to walking without support.

PROGRESSION

More vigorous exercise can be given to strengthen the quadri-ceps. A greater range of movement can be imposed on the joints, and movements entailing coordination with other joints included in the treatment. This should bring the patient to the stage where he is accustomed to the water, and ready to manage a greater degree of activity.

The exercises can be made more difficult by adding floats and by increasing the speed of performance. The following exercises may be added:

1. Half support lying—alternate hip extension.
2. Half support prone lying—alternate hip flexion.
   (In both these exercises the quadriceps work statically

but in the second one against buoyancy which will tend to flex the knee.)

3. Half support prone lying—leg movement of breast stroke.
4. Float support lying—flexion and extension patterns of leg.

Walking exercises can be varied to include walking backwards and alterations in the length of each stride.

FINAL STAGE

The aim is now to return the limb to its normal function so that the patient has a stable knee. More difficult exercises are given, with greater emphasis placed on functional and recreational activities, such as:

1. Half yard grasp standing—hip and knee flexion and extension to starting position (movement of bicycling).
2. As above with flipper added to foot.
3. Half support prone lying—leg movements of front crawl.
4. As above with flippers added to foot.
5. Lying with feet fixed under rail—hip and knee bending and stretching.

At this stage all forms of swimming provide good exercise for the legs and should be encouraged as a recreational activity. Going up and down stairs should be corrected during the middle or late stages of treatment. Group therapy can also be introduced in the middle and late stages of treatment.

The above outline can be adapted to treat other joints if the same general principles are followed.

RHEUMATOID ARTHRITIS

This condition generally starts in the smaller joints of the limbs and progresses to involve the larger ones. As many joints of the body are affected, a far more generalized treatment is usually necessary. Even though rheumatoid arthritic changes may occur in a large number of joints, they will not necessarily give trouble at the same time, and so hydrotherapy is concentrated on those joints which trouble the patient most at the time of treatment.

These patients are often more disabled than most, but are able to achieve far more during their sessions in the pool than they can on land. Many of them are confined to wheelchairs for very long periods, yet they will be able to learn to walk in the pool; pool therapy is, therefore, a source of encouragement to the more disabled rheumatoid arthritics. While difficult to move on land, in the pool these patients can be moved more easily into different starting positions, and all the affected joints can be treated in one session without causing too much stress or exhaustion.

All the symptoms previously mentioned are likely to be present, deformities of the joints being, characteristically, those of flexion. The arms tend to be held in a guarded position across the body— the shoulder in adduction and medial rotation with the elbow flexed, the forearm in the prone position and the hand and fingers flexed and in ulnar deviation. Frequently there is flexion deformity of the knee: the aim for these patients is to relieve the symptoms and to maintain as full function as possible. Rheumatoid arthritic patients usually have a good deal of pain, and this is eased in the pool by the warmth of water encompassing all the joints and by the support of the water which relieves the heaviness of the limbs resulting from muscle weakness. Wasting of the muscles, together with loss of movement, can be arrested by re-education in the pool, and, thus, deformities will be less likely to develop.

Patients are introduced to pool therapy in the subacute and chronic stages of the disease.

SUGGESTED TREATMENT

EARLY STAGE

This outline of treatment is suitable for a patient having all joints of the upper limb affected together with the knees and feet. Such a patient would probably need to be lifted into the pool by the hoist.

Sitting on a bench or stool, with the body immersed to the neck, is a good starting position, and one in which many exercises can be performed. If a greater degree of fixation seems necessary the patient can be strapped to the seat.

All exercises should be carried out in as full range as possible but within the limits of pain.

EXERCISES FOR ARMS

Sitting with elbows flexed, palms facing each other:
1. Finger bending and stretching, parting and closing.
2. Flicking water with the fingers.

3. Thumb circling.
4. Wrist bending and stretching.
5. Wrist circling.
6. Forearm—pronating and supinating.
7. Yard sitting—elbow bending and stretching.
8. Yard sitting—carry both arms to reach out and back.
9. Bend sitting—arms raising sideways and back again.
10. Bend sitting—arms raising forwards and back again.

Exercises (9) and (10) may be carried out with the elbows straight to raise the arms, but bent to take them back again as buoyancy will resist this movement.

11. Sitting—placing hands behind the neck and on the middle of the back.

LEG EXERCISES

(*a*) *Sitting with knees slightly extended:*
1. Toe bending and stretching.
2. Foot bending and stretching.
3. Foot turning in and out.
4. Foot circling.

(*b*) *Sitting:*
5. Alternate knee bending and stretching.

If the patient is severely disabled these exercises may be given in half support lying or float lying, in which relaxation is also taught.

If the patient can stand, the following exercises may be given or added later as a progression:
1. Standing—posture correction.
2. Walk standing—weight transference.
3. Stride standing—weight transference.
4. Reach grasp standing—alternate hip and knee bending and stretching.
5. Reach grasp standing—alternate hip extension.
6. Walking with support of hydrotherapist.

PROGRESSION

The same type of exercises in sitting may be continued but with the addition of floats against buoyancy and bats to alter the stream-lined effect.

ADDITIONAL EXERCISES

1. Bend sitting holding floats—double arm stretching down to side of body.
2. Yard sitting with bats in hands—carry arms to reach position: (a) bats parallel to surface; (b) bats at right angles to surface.
3. Sitting—arm movement of breast stroke.

Breast stroke movements for the legs can be taught with the patient prone on a half plinth, with the hips free. Treatment can be progressed by supporting the patient with a ring around the thorax, which enables both arm and leg movements to be performed together; once the patient is proficient all the supports can be removed. Backstroke is taught similarly.

When two or more patients are treated together recreational activities can be introduced as group therapy. For example, patients can push a ball to one another along the surface of the water using bats.

Functional activities, such as sitting down and standing up, can be performed very easily in the pool. Despite the difference in muscle work which is involved on dry land, such exercises are valuable in allowing the patient to practise the movement, and in helping to establish confidence in his ability. The patient is also taught to climb stairs, starting on the lower ones, and progressing until, with assistance, he can dispense with the hoist on entering and leaving the pool. Walking is also progressed by increasing the speed and direction of movement, and the length of step.

ANKYLOSING SPONDYLITIS

This condition is characterized by rigidity of the spine and thorax, and usually spreads to involve the hip joints and sometimes shoulders also. The age of onset is usually between 20 and 40 years, and the condition occurs mainly in men. Pool therapy is an excellent type of treatment and the patient can be encouraged to adopt swimming as a sport.

Discomfort, in the form of continual aching pain, is a fairly constant feature, with pain occurring in the muscles of the spine, hips and other affected joints. The spinal muscles, in particular, are subject to spasm which persists even after the pain has been alleviated. Spasm is responsible for much of the limitation in movement, especially in the earlier stages.

The deformity is one of flexion. Changes in the joints also contribute to the limited movement, and lead eventually to bony ankylosis.

Patients with ankylosing spondylitis will come for pool treatment at various stages of the disease. In the early stages, for patients who have pain and stiffness but no deformity, the aims are to make the back strong and mobile, and to correct posture. In addition, mobility and strength must be maintained in the hips and shoulders, and the mobility of the thorax increased. Patients in later stages will have varying degrees of deformity, as well as pain and stiffness. The deformity must be corrected, if possible, and prevented from deteriorating further.

Treatment in the pool includes exercises for all the affected joints. The patient can be taught to relax by supporting the body with floats positioned behind the head, under the back, behind the knees and ankles and under the arms. In this float support lying position correct posture can also be taught. As the deformity is one of flexion, extension exercises for the spine and hips can be done in this supported position, by pushing back against the floats and buoyancy. Shoulder exercises should be given also.

Breast stroke swimming should be taught, and the patient encouraged to practise this as it gives a good range of movement in the hips and shoulders, and uses the back extensor muscles strongly. Patients with a great deal of flexion deformity may not be able to swim in the prone position, in which case they are taught backstroke only.

Water is a particularly good medium for patients with ankylosing spondylitis as, on land, the pull of gravity tends to increase the flexion deformity, and the back extensor muscles continually go into spasm in an attempt to correct it. In water gravity is counteracted by the force of buoyancy and support given to the body. The treatment also enables breathing control to be taught in the sitting position so that the thorax expands against the surrounding pressure of the water. The patient's vital capacity can be increased by holding the breath under water, later progressing to swimming under water if the patient is capable of doing this.

SUGGESTED EXERCISES AND PROGRESSION

Float support lying

1. Breathing exercises; in this position the thorax is only partially surrounded by water, therefore meeting less resistance.
2. Relaxation using the contrast method. This may also be combined with breathing exercises.
3. Static contraction of the back muscles.
4. Gluteal and quadriceps contractions.
5. Correction of posture. This should be given throughout the treatment.
6. Head extension, pushing back into float support and water, and relaxation.
7. Head flexion from side to side.
8. Head turning from side to side, with float removed, and head supported by hydrotherapist.
9. Raising both arms to shoulder level and back.
10. Leg parting and closing.

With leg floats removed

1. Alternate leg pushing down into water and relax.
2. Progress to both legs. The hydrotherapist fixes the patient's head.
3. With knees bent to a right angle, knee parting and closing (hip rotation).

With arm floats removed

1. Pushing both arms down into water, and relax.
2. Place hands behind back and neck.

Following these, exercises can be given in standing, and walking with posture correction taught.

STRONGER EXERCISES

These may be added gradually depending on the patient's capabilities.

1-2. *Float support lying with feet under rail*, and with bats in hands. Repeat exercises (9) and (1) for arms as above, bats streamlined progressing to unstreamlined.
3. Lifting alternate arms up out of water and above head, down into water and back to side (back stroke). Given first without bats.

Lying with hydrotherapist fixing head
1. Leg movement of backstroke.
2. Trunk side flexion by moving legs.
3. With floats on feet, pushing both legs down into water, and relax.

Prone lying with arms supported on rail
1. Breast stroke movement of legs.
2. Bending both knees to chest and straightening.

Sitting
1. Breathing exercises.
2. Breast stroke movement for arms.
3. Arms in yard, trunk turning from side to side.
4. Float support lying—flexion—abduction pattern for both arms.

FINAL PROGRESSION

Lying with feet fixed under rail
1. Trunk bending from side to side.
2. Vigorous backstroke movement with arms, bats in hands. Gradually adding all swimming strokes, crawl and breast stroke with breathing control.
3. Float lying—extension patterns of back using arms or legs.

Somersaults are a useful exercise to increase movement in the spine, and to add to the patient's vital capacity. Underwater swimming can then be attempted if the patient is competent enough. While giving the patient these energetic and rather difficult exercises, the importance of relaxation and correct posture must be stressed continually.

The other conditions which will come for pool treatment are the non-articular shoulder conditions such as rotator cuff lesions. With these patients the aims of hydrotherapy are to mobilize the shoulder-joint and strengthen the muscles around it, the treatment being similar to that given for any stiff joint. Pain is eased by the warmth and buoyancy of the water and buoyancy is used first to assist, and then to resist the movement. All swimming strokes are beneficial but have to be modified according to the patient's ability to swim.

For rheumatic conditions, pool therapy is given in conjunction with dry land exercises, and should enable the patient to progress extremely well.

8

The Treatment of Neurological Disorders

POOL THERAPY is used extensively in the treatment of many neurological disorders. The warmth and support of the water helps to relieve some of the patient's symptoms, and a graduated progression of exercises is of value to patients whose muscles are weak or paralysed. As well as giving the patient support and freedom of movement, the warm water enables the hydrotherapist to move him more easily than on land. As with other conditions, these factors improve both the patient's confidence and his morale.

The aims of treatment for neurological conditions are to reduce muscle spasm, to re-educate paralysed muscles, to strengthen weak muscles, to maintain joint mobility, and to re-educate for functional activities. The relative importance of these aims, however, will vary with the different conditions to be treated.

SIGNS AND SYMPTOMS

Firstly, the common signs and symptoms which can be helped by pool therapy must be considered.

Weakness or paralysis. A patient is said to be paralysed if he is unable to perform voluntary movement. When the upper motor neurone is affected, the patient is unable to initiate the voluntary movement, though the muscles remain capable of contracting. The condition is known as paralysis of movement. If the lower motor neurone is affected, the patient is able to initiate the movement, but the final common pathway is damaged and the ability of the muscles to contract is lost; this is known as paralysis of muscles. The lack of use leads eventually to muscle atrophy, which will hamper

7

recovery when the capacity for voluntary movement begins to return.

The pool provides an excellent medium for the re-education of voluntary muscle power. When the muscle is very weak, active exercises are given, using buoyancy as an assistance. As power increases, buoyancy is used as a support, and with further recovery, as a form of resistance.

This fine progression is invaluable where the muscles retain little power but a good range of movement, and with recovery, the difficulty of the exercise can be increased very gradually. A muscle graded as 1 on the Oxford scale* can perform movement with buoyancy assisting; as the flicker of movement becomes stronger the exercise can be progressed, using buoyancy as a support; by the time that the muscle is graded as 2, it can work against buoyancy. As the power increases to grade 3 and then to grade 4, so the resistance of buoyancy is increased by lengthening the weight arm of the lever and by adding floats.

Alteration in tone. Tone may be increased, decreased or lost completely. Increase in tone is due either to lack of inhibition of anterior horn cell activity, or to irritation of the excitatory part of the reticular formation. The former is found in upper motor neurone lesions; for example, the spasticity of hemiplegia (see below). This is characterized by an increased resistance to passive movement, which is maximal at the beginning of movement. The spasticity predominates in the flexors of the upper limb and in the extensors of the lower limb.

When the excitatory part of the reticular formation is irritated, tone is increased in all muscles in the affected part of the body, as in Parkinson's disease. With this increase in tone, resistance to passive movement is maintained throughout the whole range of movement, and is termed 'rigidity'.

Decrease in tone, or flaccidity, results from decreased excitability of the anterior horn cells. Therefore, disease or damage affecting the final common pathway leads to decreased or lost tone, as in anterior poliomyelitis and peripheral nerve injuries. As a result of

* *The Oxford Scale of Muscle Power* (on land)

0 = No contraction	3 = Movement against gravity
1 = A flicker of movement	4 = Movement against gravity
2 = Movement with gravity	and resistance
eliminated	5 = Normal

the reduction in tone, voluntary movement is either lost or impaired, and as these atrophic muscles have little protection they are damaged easily.

During pool therapy, the warmth of the water helps to relieve spasticity, even if the relief is only temporary. However, as the spasm diminishes, passive movements can be given in a greater range and with less discomfort to the patient. In this way joint range can be maintained. When treating a patient with strong adductor spasm in the legs, a marked difference is noticed, even after 10 minutes in the pool, when an increase in the range of abduction is evident.

The passive movements must be given slowly and rhythmically; as the limb is supported by the water—with or without the assistance of floats—the hydrotherapist's attention can be devoted to the performance of the movement. The chief difficulty is to obtain a stable fixation both for patient and hydrotherapist. The most stable position for the patient is to be strapped on to a plinth fixed to the rail of the pool. The hydrotherapist braces herself by taking a wide stance, but in some instances a second hydrotherapist may be needed to fix the other limb.

Formation of contracture and loss of joint movement. Contractures and deformities hamper recovery of voluntary power. They often occur in diseases affecting upper or lower motor neurones, and result from the contracture of fibrosed joint structures, or muscle imbalance leading to adaptive contractures of the muscles. This is seen in the typical hemiplegic arm or in contracture of the calf muscles following paralysis of the anterior tibial muscles. The resulting stiff joints hamper voluntary movement, and they occur wherever contractures have formed or where there is loss of movement in a joint.

If voluntary muscle power is absent, passive movements are used to prevent contractures and to maintain joint range. A full range movement is essential, but if this is limited by pain, the movement should be carried through as great a range as possible. If contractures have developed, gentle stretching is given within the limits of pain, the warmth of the water making the procedure far less painful than on dry land. As soon as voluntary power begins to return, active exercises replace the passive movements, and are given with the assistance at the limits of the range.

Loss of coordination. Coordination of movement depends on

the correct correlation of all the pathways of the nervous system, and the resulting harmonious working of muscle groups. If any of the pathways are damaged incoordination develops and can result in muscle imbalance, muscle weakness or spasticity. There are two other types of incoordination, namely sensory and cerebellar ataxia. In sensory ataxia the patient is unaware of the position of his limbs in space unless he uses his vision to see where they are. In cerebellar ataxia the controlling influence of the cerebellum is lost, hence the inability to perform a smooth, purposeful movement.

Although the incoordination associated with muscle weakness and spasticity responds to hydrotherapy, patients with sensory or cerebellar ataxia seem to derive little benefit. While a normal person finds it hard to retain his balance in water—partly due to buoyancy and partly to the turbulance created by movement—the ataxic patient has even more difficulty, which is intensified by the effect of refraction distorting the limbs under water.

Training in coordination is started with the patient lying on a plinth; rhythmic stabilizations are given to the trunk, and progression is made through sitting to standing. Once the patient can stand upright, the treatment can be made more difficult by using turbulence and encouraging the patient to stand still in one place. When this has been mastered, the patient can be taught to walk and turn in the water. Again turbulence is used as a progression. Exercises changing the position of the arms and head are given in sitting and, finally, in standing positions. As soon as the patient has sufficient control of his balance both in sitting and standing, ball games can be introduced.

Circulatory impairment. Lack of voluntary movement and disturbance of the conductivity of the sympathetic fibres of the nervous system leads to stagnation of blood and failure of the sebaceous and sweat glands to function normally. The skin becomes blue and shiny, there is lack of sweat and the hairs tend to fall out. The muscle fibres decrease in size and gradually become fibrosed.

During hydrotherapy the warmth of the water dilates superficial blood vessels, producing a faint reddening of the skin; this vaso-dilatation improves the blood supply, and thus helps to prevent impaired nutrition of the skin. Great care must be taken in handling patients with trophic changes; this is particularly important in the water, because the skin breaks down easily and is slow to heal. The deep circulation can be helped by movement—active when possible, otherwise passive movements.

The pressure of the water is directly proportional to its depth. If an oedematous limb is suspended in water, the pressure exerted on the foot is greater than on the thigh. The resulting difference in lateral pressure forces the oedema upwards. The improvement in circulation is clearly evident in the change in colour of the limbs during treatment. Before treatment the limb is blue and congested, but afterwards has a much healthier pink colour.

Pain. Pain hampers voluntary movement, and occurs for several reasons. The usual causes are stretching of the contractures during treatment, active inflammation in the nerve sheaths or meninges, and the accumulation of metabolites as a result of impaired circulation. Both the warmth and the support of the water help to relieve pain and the warmth also improves the circulation. As the pain is eased care must be taken not to overstretch the contractures during passive movements, as this will intensify the pain.

HEMIPLEGIA

A paralysis of one side of the body, which may also involve the face of the same or opposite side, is known as hemiplegia. Initially the limbs are flaccid, and the patient may be unconscious, but many cases progress to a second stage—the onset of spasticity. It is at this stage that the patient will start pool treatment.

The patient is allowed into the pool when his blood pressure has returned to a reasonable level and when further damage by haemorrhage is no longer likely; generally this would be 3 to 4 weeks after the cerebral accident.

The patient is lowered slowly into the pool by the hoist, and is watched carefully for signs of distress. A momentary rise in blood pressure will occur owing to vasoconstriction as he enters the pool, but is followed almost immediately by vasodilatation, causing a fall in blood pressure. The hydrotherapist must stay with the patient at all times, continuing to watch for signs of distress.

The aim of the first treatment, which lasts 5 to 10 minutes, is to accustom the patient to the water. For this initial session he is strapped on to a plinth, and is encouraged to relax and become used to the feeling of weightlessness. Breathing exercises may be given.

As voluntary movements return, selective spasticity tends to develop, causing the arm to be flexed, adducted and medially rotated, while the knee and ankle of the lower limb are extended. The shoulder-joint is particularly prone to stiffness. Passive movements to both arm and leg are given, in as full a range as possible, particular care being necessary to prevent the shoulder from becoming stiff and to obtain dorsi-flexion of the ankle. The movements are performed with the patient supported on a plinth, and should be carried out slowly and rhythmically. They are given within the limits of pain, as any forced movement will result in increased spasticity. Exercises should be carried out in mass patterns to help the patient to remember the normal pattern of movement, and the patient should be encouraged to think about the movement as it is carried out by the hydrotherapist. Exercises to reduce spasticity by using reflex inhibitory postures and shaking the limbs can be combined with passive movements.

The fine grading of resistance by buoyancy is utilized in the re-education of voluntary movement. The undamaged pathways must be made to work as hard as possible, by giving maximum resistance to the muscles supplied by these pathways—the use of floats and maximum manual resistance can be used to great advantage. The patient is given general exercises for the affected arm and leg, lying on a plinth or on body floats progressing to sitting on a seat, and then to standing and holding on to the parallel bars or to the hydrotherapist for support. If the patient has a flail knee, a polythene back splint can be bandaged on to it to prevent the knee from giving way. The patient then transfers his weight from side to side, and forwards and backwards.

Once he has mastered standing, re-education in the walking pattern is started. Spasticity and weak muscles often hamper movement so that the patient tends to drag his leg and swing it forward through an abduction arc. The buoyancy of the water will help to flex the hips and knee, and counteract dragging of the leg. First he is asked to 'Bend the knee', 'Straighten the knee', 'Put the heel down' and 'Rock forward on to your toes', this being emphasized as he begins to walk either between parallel bars or holding on to the hydrotherapist for support. (It is better for the hydrotherapist to stand in front of the patient, and let him put his hands on her shoulders, than to walk beside him.) As walking improves, support can be reduced to a single rail, and eventually this support, too, can be removed.

Swimming plays a great part in the re-education of coordination. Prowess at swimming depends greatly on the amount of voluntary power and the patient's ability to swim. At first, he will tend to swim in circles because of the unequal pull of the unaffected arm and leg. As he improves, this tendency becomes less apparent, and the patient finds encouragement in his ability to perform some recreational activity. The type of swimming stroke will depend on the patient's previous swimming ability. Generally, it is easier to start on the back and progress to swimming face downwards.

Games in which various sizes of ball are pushed through the water are used to re-educate balance, and are given in sitting or standing positions, depending on the ability of the patient to balance.

As on dry land, functional activities play a great part in the rehabilitation of the hemiplegic patient. He should practise standing up and sitting down, since these motions are made much easier by the effect of buoyancy, and help the patient to remember the pattern of movement. Climbing stairs is also included in the scheme of treatment. At first, only the lower steps, where the effect of buoyancy is maximal, are attempted, but as the patient becomes stronger he can tackle the higher steps as well.

TRAUMATIC PARAPLEGIA

Paralysis of both lower limbs follows dislocation, at certain levels, of the thoracic or lumbar vertebrae, possibly with fracture, causing damage to the spinal cord or corda equina. If the lesion is above the level of the first thoracic vertebra the arms will be involved also, causing a quadriplegia. Any lesion above the fifth thoracic vertebra may cause respiratory impairment. If the lesion is below the first lumbar vertebra the cauda equina is involved, and the lesion is of the lower motor neurone type; if above, an upper motor neurone lesion will result.

Recovery depends on the extent of the damage: with complete severance of the cord no voluntary power will return, but if the severance is partial or if symptoms are due to pressure some return of voluntary power can be expected.

A patient will be given hydrotherapy when the fracture or dislocation has consolidated and provided that his vital capacity is not below 1500 cm^3. He will suffer from some degree of incontinence, so his bladder must be emptied before entering the pool, and it must be ascertained that his bowels have been emptied that day. To prevent any contamination of the water, the level of chlorination can be stepped up or treatment given at the end of the day.

At first the patient is lowered into the pool by hoist. As he improves he can be taught to use a pulley, and swing himself into the pool. The hydrotherapist must, however, always be at hand to give help and to prevent accidents.

Passive movements to all joints of the lower limbs are given with the patient lying on a plinth. Any voluntary power that remains is strengthened by the usual exercises appropriate to the area.

Exercises are given for the arms and trunk, the arm exercises being taken at first with the patient lying on the plinth, and later, in the sitting position. Particular attention is paid to strengthening the shoulder extensors and adductors and the elbow extensors, as these are the arm muscles needed for crutch walking. Resistance is used in the form of bats and floats. Trunk exercises to strengthen all muscle groups are given in lying and sitting positions. Fixation of the trunk, by using the arms, helps in strengthening both arm and trunk muscles; the patient can swing his legs from side to side, in this way strengthening the trunk side flexors and the latissimus dorsi. The exercise is progressed by adding floats and rings.

Balance will depend on the site of the lesion, and is less affected if the abdominal muscles are not involved, as with lesions occurring below the thoracic vertebrae. Vision plays a great part in maintaining balance, and a mirror at the side of the pool is helpful to unsteady patients. At first balance is taught in float lying, with rhythmic stabilization to the trunk and pelvis; progression is to sitting and, finally, to standing. Turbulence of the water is used as a progression in sitting or standing exercises, and further progression is by using simple unilateral and bilateral arm exercises. The exercises then proceed from sitting with support, through sitting without support, and, eventually, to ball games in unsupported sitting.

When the patient can sit unaided he can begin to learn to stand. He is taught to stand and lock his knee joints by extending the hips. If he cannot do this, a polythene back splint can be bandaged to the knees for support. Standing is taught first in the parallel bars, holding on to the therapist or to rail of the pool. The hydrotherapist stands facing the patient and supports the pelvis, while the patient rests his hands on her shoulders or forearms. The degree of proficiency in walking again depends on the level of the lesion; with lower lesions the use of the abdominal muscles is retained, but this is not so with the higher level lesions when only the latissimus dorsi muscles are working. If the patient has the use of his abdominal muscles a swing-to gait, and later a swing-through gait are taught. When the abdominal muscles are paralysed the patient is taught to hitch his legs forward, using the latissimus dorsi.

Swimming is taught from the beginning, when floating on the back will be the easiest position for the patient. The legs will lie lower in the water than the rest of the body. Sculling with the arms is taught first, then the arms are brought slowly up and out of the water, and down quickly through the water, thus providing the propelling force. Progression is made from double-arm back crawl to alternate-arm back crawl. Swimming in the prone position will depend on the ability of the patient to extend his neck. Patients with lower lesions will be able to swim in this position but those with higher cervical lesions will have difficulty; they can be taught, however, provided the hydrotherapist stays with the patient, and can turn him over whenever he needs to breathe.

MULTIPLE SCLEROSIS

This is a chronic disease of unknown aetiology, affecting the brain and spinal cord. The signs and symptoms depend on the site of the lesion, but can be divided into three basic groups—upper motor neurone, cerebellar and sensory. The groups are not clearly defined, however, as most patients show mixed signs with one group predominating. Patients in the cerebellar and sensory groups gain less benefit from pool therapy than those in whom upper motor neurone symptoms predominate.

As many of the patients, particularly the advanced cases, suffer from incontinence, care must be taken to see that the bladder is emptied before treatment.

The aims of treatment are similar to those for the hemiplegic patient, and include reduction of spasticity, prevention of contractures, and re-education of voluntary power and functional activities. In advanced cases, the pool is of great value in relieving the pain arising from spasticity, and since this may be the only place where the patient is able to relax and be relatively free from pain, the hydrotherapist may well find she has an eager and cooperative patient.

Treatment is divided into early and advanced stages.

EARLY STAGE

Passive movements are given to prevent contractures from developing. Active exercises then follow, using the manual resistance or the resistance of buoyancy and floats whenever possible. As the condition is progressive, the patient may become chairbound, so the emphasis is to strengthen the arms, making him as independent as possible. In addition, general arm and trunk exercises are given, with particular emphasis on the latissimus dorsi, the elbow extensors and all the trunk muscles. Exercises for the legs are introduced to maintain mobility and strength. Functional activities such as walking, climbing stairs, sitting down and standing up can all be given in water. The relief of weight by buoyancy makes it possible for these patients to walk in the water when muscle weakness makes this impossible on land. The morale of the patient can be raised by recreational activities such as swimming and ball games.

ADVANCED STAGE

By this stage the patient is probably in considerable pain from contractures that have developed due to spasticity and muscle imbalance. Relaxation is encouraged with the patient completely supported in the water by floats. The warmth of the water and the support aids this relaxation, and passive movements and stretching can then be given. Any remaining voluntary movement should be encouraged, but care should be taken not to overtire the patient. By now the patient will probably be completely chairbound and unable to walk, even in the pool. The visit to the pool provides an outing for such patients to look forward to, and this, apart from the beneficial effects of treatment, is of great psychological value.

SUGGESTED EXERCISES

The following are suggested exercises for a patient with an upper motor neurone lesion affecting both legs and with minimal weakness of arms. These are a guide to the type of exercises that might be given, selection depending on the requirements of individual patients.

Exercises (1)–(7) are given with the patient lying on a half plinth, with floats at the knees and elbows for exercises (1) and (2), and at the knees only for exercises (6) and (7).

Half support lying
1. General relaxation and posture correction.
2. Passive movements to all joints of lower limb.
3. Alternate hip extension—add floats.
4. Alternate knee bending and stretching with manual resistance.
5. Double foot bending and stretching with manual resistance.
6. Double arm raising sideways to yard and back—add bats.
7. Double arm pushing down into water and back—add bats.

Heave grasp half support lying
8. Double leg swinging to alternate sides.
9. Back arching and relax.

Sitting
10. Rhythmic stabilizations.
11. Throwing ball to hydrotherapist.
12. Sitting → standing → sitting.
13. Reach grasp standing—alternate hip extension.
14. Walking forwards and sideways.
15. Float support lying—arms as for back stroke.
16. Float support prone lying—arms as for breast stroke.

PARKINSON'S DISEASE

This is a degenerative disease of the extrapyramidal system, and usually develops first between 50 and 65 years of age. Degenerative changes occur in the basal ganglia, and the disease is characterized by tremor and muscular rigidity, with slowing and weakening of voluntary movements. The condition is slowly progressive and eventually the patient may become completely immobile.

Hydrotherapy can help to relieve pain caused by rigidity, and relaxation exercises, with the body supported by floats, help to counteract the flexed posture that develops. Constant emphasis must be put on 'letting the limbs go' and floating in the water.

The patient is thus able to relax in a good position, gaining some relief from pain. The warmth of the water also helps to reduce both rigidity and tremor.

Contractures resulting from rigidity can be prevented by using rhythmical, slow passive movements. Such movements, together with the warmth of the water, help to increase the circulation, thereby aiding the removal of metabolites which are irritant and cause pain.

To gain stronger and quicker voluntary movements, general active exercises are given. Large range movements for the arms and legs are given easily in the water which provides an excellent medium for free movement. Pool therapy is also valuable for walking re-education as buoyancy makes it easier to move the legs, aiding hip and knee flexion, thus preventing the shuffling gait which is so characteristic of the condition. Swimming will help co-ordination.

The treatment of these patients requires a great deal of patience and understanding, and care must be taken to encourage them when possible, not to overtire them, and not to hurry them along.

ACUTE POLIOMYELITIS

This acute infectious disease is caused by a virus which has an affinity for the anterior horn cells of the spinal cord and the brain stem. Acute poliomyelitis presents a classic clinical picture of a febrile illness resembling influenza, followed by muscular paralysis which varies in extent from patient to patient, but is widespread at first. The paralysis is of the lower motor neurone type, with flaccid muscles and loss of tendon reflexes. After the acute phase, there is residual, and usually asymmetrical, paralysis of certain muscle groups. The affected muscles are tested out of the water and charted on the Oxford scale. The muscles are also tested in the water using the following modified scale:

0 = No contraction
1 = Contraction with buoyancy assisting
2 = Contraction with buoyancy eliminated
2+ = Contraction against buoyancy
3 = Contraction against buoyancy (at speed)
4 = Contraction against buoyancy (light float)
5 = Contraction against buoyancy (large float)

The recovery rate is rapid during the first 6 months. If a muscle has no flicker after 6 months, it is unlikely to regain movement, but any flicker at all indicates a possible recovery of voluntary power. After 2 years the muscles may show no further increase in power, but its function may continue to improve for up to 7 years.

The patient is allowed into the pool after the acute stage has subsided and the temperature has been back to normal for a week. Patients with respiratory involvement are allowed in the pool provided the vital capacity is more than 1500 cm³. As there is a long period of recovery the patient must be encouraged at all times and his interest maintained; this is particularly important in the treatment of children.

Because of their poor circulation, the affected limbs are often cold and blue, and the warmth of the water does much to improve the blood flow; it also helps to warm the muscles and so enables them to contract more easily. Full range of movement must be maintained in all joints and helps prevent contractures and maintain the circulation. Passive movements are used where the muscles are too weak to produce movement.

General strengthening exercises are given to unaffected muscles, and maximal resistance using mass movement patterns are of great value. The fine progression of resistance provided by buoyancy gives an ideal method for strengthening weakened muscles, but great care must be taken not to tire them in the early stages. Trick movements should be avoided until there is no hope of full recovery.

The psychological benefit of pool therapy cannot be stressed too strongly, especially in the treatment of younger patients. When the patient can see that some movement is present, no matter how slight, he is encouraged and will work harder to achieve even better results.

The scheme of treatment will vary from patient to patient, but a carefully graded progression is used for all affected muscles, the starting point and rate of progression depending on the individual patient.

Recreational activities play a great part in maintaining the patient's morale, as well as generally strengthening his muscles and keeping him mobile. All the swimming strokes provide valuable exercise, from the simplest sculling movements to the more advanced breast stroke and crawl. Competitive games such as swimming are to be encouraged, provided that the patients are at more or less the same stage of recovery. Once the patient can swim safely by himself, he should be encouraged to go to the local baths, or to join a swimming club, though he must be warned of the difference in temperature, for unless he is able to keep moving, the colder water will cause discomfort and may therefore discourage him from further effort.

All functional activities previously mentioned should be included in the scheme of treatment.

POLYNEURITIS

This condition affects the brain stem and many peripheral nerves, and it is usually symmetrical, resulting in widespread muscle weakness, pain and sensory loss. The condition of the patient usually deteriorates rapidly, then shows a slow improvement, many patients recovering completely.

Bed rest is essential in the early stages, with careful positioning of the limbs; passive movements must be carried out several times a day.

Pool therapy can begin with the first signs of recovery, and is very similar to the treatment for acute poliomyelitis. The main aims are to prevent contractures, to maintain the circulation and to build up muscular power, using the fine grades of progression possible in the water.

PERIPHERAL NERVE LESIONS

Three main types of nerve lesions can occur:

1. *Neurotmesis*—the most serious—in which the nerve is completely severed. Suture is essential, and even then, recovery is incomplete because of the scar tissue which tends to obstruct and misdirect the nerve fibres into the distal neurolemma sheath. The prognosis is poor.

2. *Axonotomesis*, in which the axons degenerate but the supporting neurolemma remains intact. As the nerve fibres take time to regenerate, the affected muscles become paralysed, but eventually recover. The prognosis is good.

3. *Neuropraxia*, in which there is a block in the conduction

of nerve impulses due to pressure or bruising, but no degeneration of nerve fibres. Recovery is quick and the prognosis good.

The main effects of these lesions are loss of muscle power, impaired circulation, stiff joints, deformity and trophic changes. The pool is useful in maintaining the circulation, thereby preventing trophic changes and stiff joints, and it facilitates the re-education of the returning muscle power.

The patient with neurotmesis is allowed into the pool when the sutures have been removed and when recovery from the initial shock of injury has worn off. With all types of lesion care must be taken not to damage the skin, and the area of the lesion should be dried carefully after treatment.

Passive movements to the affected joints prevent deformities and, together with the warmth of the water, maintain the circulation; warmth also makes the movements more comfortable. Once voluntary power has recovered, active exercises can be introduced, using buoyancy as an assistance, as a support and, finally, as a resistance, and suitable arm or leg patterns all indicated by the lesion.

BRACHIAL PLEXUS LESION

The lesion may be complete or partial, upper trunk lesions being the most common. In complete lesions all muscles of the upper limb except the trapezius are paralysed, and sensation is completely lost. Partial lesions of the upper trunk affect the muscles of the shoulder and the elbow flexors, while lesions of the lower trunk affect the muscles of the hand. If the lesion is complete the arm may have to be amputated, but in partial lesions a combination of surgery, splinting and physical therapy help to restore function.

Pool therapy is often used in the treatment of partial lesions, and begins as soon as the initial shock has worn off. Passive movements to the affected joints can be given satisfactorily with the patient lying and supported by floats. By using the fine progression of buoyancy, voluntary power can be re-educated. Functional activities involving the use of the whole arm must be encouraged.

The following is an outline of progressive treatment for a patient suffering from a partial brachial plexus lesion:

Particular care must be taken to ensure that the shoulder is completely covered by the water, and the patient should sit on a graded bench or be instructed to bend his knees so that his shoulders are submerged. A common fault with all shoulder injuries is reversed scapulo-humeral rhythm, but if a mirror is placed at the side of the pool the patient can watch the movement and correct any faults.

EARLY STAGE

1. Support lying—passive movements to all joints of arm.
2. Sitting—posture correction, with emphasis on the level of the shoulder girdle.
3. Yard sitting—elbow bend and stretch.
4. Sitting—arms lifting sidewards (returned to starting position by hydrotherapist).
5. Forearm support inclined standing—arm lifting forwards (returned to starting position by hydrotherapist).
6. Sitting—arm lifting backwards (returned to starting position by hydrotherapist).
7. Sitting—shoulder shrug and relax.
8. Reach prone lying (across stretcher)—arms lifting backwards.
9. Sitting, pushing small ball through the water to the hydrotherapist.

Exercises (3), (4), (5), (6), (8) and (9) can be progressed by using bats and increasing the speed of performance.

LATER STAGE

1. Support lying—arm lifting sidewards and back.
2. Alternate side support lying—uppermost arm swinging upwards and back.
3. Support lying—arm pushing backwards and up.
4. Yard support lying—arms pushing backwards and up.
5. Sitting—arm raising sideways and down; with small bat → larger bat.
6. Forearm support incline standing—arm swinging forwards and backwards; with a small bat.
7. Sitting—movements of breast stroke.
8. Yard sitting—pushing a float across the water; with small bat.
9. Sitting—placing the hand behind neck, then behind the back.

10. Reach sitting—arm pushing downwards and back—add bat.
11. Float support lying—sculling.
12. Swimming—breast stroke, front crawl, back crawl.
13. Float lying—arm movement patterns.

This scheme of treatment is intended only as a guide. The progression will vary with each patient and will be accompanied with treatment in the gymnasium. The final stages of rehabilitation will be carried out in the gymnasium and swimming pool only.

9

The Treatment of Orthopaedic Conditions

WATER is used extensively in the treatment of orthopaedic conditions. Because of its buoyancy, support and warmth, water provides both a means of achieving relaxation and exercise, and is a medium in which re-education, independence and rehabilitation can be gained.

When treating orthopaedic conditions the emphasis is mainly on re-education. With a few exceptions the patient has probably sustained injury or undergone orthopaedic surgery, and re-education of muscle power, movement, coordination and functional abilities is essential. In many instances, re-education can begin early in treatment, because the buoyancy of the water enables the patient to bear weight and to move affected muscles so much more easily than he could do on land. For example, in the case of joints above and below a comparatively recent fracture sight, greater range of movement can be expected in water than on land. This great advantage of early ambulation and fuller movements enables the patient to gain confidence and independence quickly, while relatively normal patterns of movement, and the pathways to and from the brain can be maintained. Pool therapy should always be given in conjunction with, and supplementary to, dry land treatments.

SIGNS AND SYMPTOMS

Orthopaedic conditions suitable for pool therapy may be characterized by pain, bruising, oedema and tenderness, limitation of joint movement, muscle weakness, loss of coordination, limping and deformity.

1. *Pain.* This varies in degree according to the site affected, and the time since injury or surgery. Although acute pain may have been eased by previous fixation, it may still be severe. It is essential, therefore, to take care when moving the patient and, in particular, the affected limbs or joint.

2. *Bruising, oedema and tenderness.* These symptoms are especially characteristic of fractures and dislocations. Bruising will disappear gradually after fixation but oedema may be persistent.

3. *Limitation of joint movement.* This may be due to injury, previous fixation or traction. In some cases a joint that was unaffected originally may become involved: hip surgery can result in a stiff knee joint, and an elbow injury may limit movement in the shoulder. Movement may also be limited by pain, muscle spasm or weakness.

4. *Muscle weakness.* Muscle weakness will naturally occur if a part has been wholly or partially immobilized in plaster or by traction. If the patient suffers severe pain, he may be unable to contract the affected muscles, even isometrically, and wasting occurs because of inactivity. Protective muscle spasm also leads to immobility and consequent muscle weakness; for example, spasm of the hamstring muscles often leads to quadriceps inhibition. Inability to complete a full-range movement because of a stiff joint means that the muscles are not used to this full capacity, and weakness is the inevitable result.

5. *Incoordination.* This is generally co-existent with muscle spasm or weakness, and stiffness of the joint. If movement in one knee joint is limited through immobilization, an incoordinated bicycling movement will result. Other movements of this type— reversed scapulo-humeral rhythm, for example—must be corrected from the first treatment so that the development of 'trick' movements is prevented.

6. *Limping.* A limp may be due to limited movement of the ankle, knee or hip joints, pain and muscle weakness. True or apparent shortening of a limb also causes limping. The cause of the limp should be investigated, treated and corrected. True shortening of a limb can be rectified by giving the patient a weighted, built-up shoe to wear in the pool. The other causes of limping, especially weakness of the trunk muscles, may upset the patient's balance, and re-education of balance and strengthening of the

affected muscles may be necessary before walking exercises can be begun.

7. *Deformity*. This may be due to untreated chronic conditions, or to pain and muscle spasm or weakness after trauma or surgery, or to muscle atrophy caused by long-term splintage or fixation.

8. *Injury to other structures*. In many fractures and dislocations secondary injury may occur in the soft tissues, such as nerves, tendons and muscles. These may require suturing, transplanting or re-siting. The treatment of such complications, as well as treatment of the primary injury, will frequently be given by the hydrotherapist.

PRINCIPLES OF TREATMENT

The aims of treatment are to increase and maintain joint mobility; to strengthen weakened muscles, thereby preventing deformity; to improve posture, balance, coordination and gait, and to encourage functional activities and independence.

JOINT MOBILITY

With the decrease in pain resulting from muscle relaxation in the pool, a corresponding increase in joint range and activity can be expected. Exercises are selected to increase and maintain joint mobility according to the patient's disabilities, capabilities and age. The joints above and below the affected area must also be treated. The patient's range of movement is assessed in the buoyancy supported position. In the early stages of treatment, exercises are performed with buoyancy assisting the moving part, and in the greatest possible range within the limits of pain. 'Hold-relax' techniques can be used, with buoyancy again assisting movement in the new range. For example, with the patient in the bend-sitting position, the shoulder adductors work against strong resistance, but when he relaxes, shoulder abduction can be given with buoyancy assisting the movement. When some movement has been gained the exercises are repeated, with buoyancy to support the moving part; as further progress is made, buoyancy can be used to resist the movement. Floats and other forms of progression can be used at every stage, the joint being moved several times in every direction. Coordinated movements involving the affected part should be included in the treatment, with swimming and other general activities being introduced as soon as the patient is able to cope with them.

WEAKENED MUSCLES AND THE PREVENTION OF DEFORMITY

Muscle strength can be promoted and, therefore, the final degrees of mobility gained, by using a graduated progression of exercises such as the special pool techniques described in Germany, and later developed in Switzerland, by Dr Zin. Modified facilitation techniques are adapted to the patient's needs, the true diagonal being eliminated so that the limb can remain submerged. As a resisted movement takes place the body passes through the water, and the patient will overcome not only the manual resistance offered by the hydrotherapist but also that of the water.

POSTURE, BALANCE AND GAIT

Postural correction may be necessary after injury, as acquired defects can result from poor positioning or awkward stance. Exercises may be given to strengthen the trunk muscles, and, more important, the patient must be reminded continually to correct his posture. Correction may be given in lying, sitting and standing positions. Re-education of balance is begun sitting and progressed to standing. Stabilization exercises are necessary, so that the patient can learn to adjust himself to various positions, and overcome the upthrust of buoyancy.

FUNCTIONAL ACTIVITIES AND INDEPENDENCE

As soon as range and muscle power have developed sufficiently, functional activities can be encouraged. By this time the patient will have discovered that in water his capabilities are increased, and he will have gained some confidence. As he learns to move freely in water, rejecting the help of bars and other support, his confidence will increase still further. Ball games are especially useful for those with upper limb conditions. Swimming is an excellent functional activity that facilitates coordination and provides strong muscle work and joint movement for the whole body, and is valuable in almost every case. Various swimming strokes can be used to exercise particular muscles.

In the later stages of rehabilitation the emphasis is on achieving the maximum muscle power and joint range possible, and every effort should be made to achieve at least as good a function as before the injury. Treatment should be concentrated therefore on disabilities and functional requirements in particular. When rehabilitation in the pool is complete, final re-education must take place on land so that the patient can adjust himself to the force of gravity in his normal environment.

Conditions that respond well to pool therapy include (a) arthroplasty, synovectomy, spinal fusion and similar surgical procedures; (b) chronic disabilities such as spondylolithesis; (c) fractures and dislocations; (d) soft tissue injuries and tendon transplants; and (e) amputations.

In the following outlines, the times suggested for pool treatment, both initially and within a specific scheme, are only approximate indications. In every case, mobilization and progression of treatment will be as the surgeon directs.

HYDROTHERAPY FOLLOWING SURGERY OF THE LOWER LIMB

THE HIP

With the exception of arthrodesis, all types of hip surgery aim to provide a mobile, pain-free hip and to construct a suitable weight-bearing joint. Surgery commonly follows trauma or osteoarthritis of the hip. Various surgical techniques are performed.

Arthroplasty. Replacement arthroplasty is usually indicated where movements of more than one joint are restricted, for example, the lumbar spine or the opposite hip. The patient is usually middle aged or elderly. Various procedures using different forms of prostheses may be carried out, some (e.g. Austin Moore and McKee arthroplasties) requiring no traction post-operatively, the patient being treated in the pool approximately 3 to 4 weeks after operation. Cup arthroplasty involves a period of 3 to 6 weeks in traction post-operatively, after which pool therapy is started. Similarly, excision arthroplasty (Girdlestone's pseudo-arthrosis) requires a period of traction. Thus, while the treatment for all patients will follow the same lines, pool therapy may be delayed in some cases for several weeks.

Osteotomy. Abduction osteotomy employing McMurray techniques may be treated 3 to 4 weeks after surgery, and osteotomies using the Muller compression techniques as early as 2 weeks after operation.

Arthrodesis. The patient is usually young, but as a long period of immobilization is customary pool treatment will not begin for 8 to 12 weeks after operation.

The following is a guide to treatment after arthroplasty and osteotomy:

EARLY STAGE (3 to 6 weeks after operation)
Entry to pool is by the hoist and the patient is treated for 20 to 30 minutes. Exercises using buoyancy as a support are given in fixed or semi-fixed positions. Lateral rotation should be avoided at this stage, the main aims being to gain mobility and increase the power of the extensors and abductors of the hip. Exercises for the knees are included as knee joints may have stiffened during traction. The spine is also exercised, particularly in patients with osteo-arthritis who may have developed a compensatory lordosis.

Half support lying
   1. Leg parting and closing.
   2. Bending the knees to 90° and, keeping them together, parting the ankles (medial rotation).
   3. Hip extension.

Half support side lying
   1. Knee bending and stretching.
   2. Hip bending and stretching with straight knee: repeat the movement against manual resistance on extension.

The above may be progressed by adding floats or flippers to the moving part, or by increasing the speed of movement.

LATER STAGES (5 to 10 weeks)
Some increase in muscle strength and joint mobility will have been gained. Combined hip and knee movements are encouraged, against the resistance of buoyancy, and lateral rotation is permitted. The patient is able to stand, and re-education of balance, walking, and posture is begun. Entering the pool by hoist is progressed to entering by the stairs.

Half support lying
1. Adduction of under leg.
2. Float at knee—hip extension.
3. Knee bending and stretching.
4. Knees bent to 90°—knee parting keeping ankles together (lateral rotation).
5. Support lying with feet fixed under the rail of the pool—bending and stretching the hips and knees.
6. Reach grasp standing—affected hip and knee flexed and a float round the ankle. Straighten leg, bracing the knee back.
7. Side inclined standing affected leg uppermost—adduction of uppermost leg.
8. Float lying—leg patterns of movement.

Balance re-education. The patient sits, if possible, between submerged parallel bars. Rhythmic stabilizations for the trunk are given, followed by pelvic stabilizations in stride standing, and then walk standing. The patient can use the bars as a support when first standing. Weight transference is taught, again in stride standing, then in walk standing. Standing up from the sitting position should be attempted, for although this movement is assisted, many patients find it difficult to control.

Posture. Correct posture prevents deformity and ensures equal distribution of body weight. Posture can be taught in sitting, and then in standing positions and entails constant correction of the pelvic tilt.

Walking. Side steps are taken first, the patient holding the pool rail or being supported by the hydrotherapist. Once he has achieved even steps, the patient can attempt to walk unaided. As soon as side stepping has been mastered, forward and, later, backward walking is introduced. These can be begun within parallel bars, if available. The hands are moved along the bars as they would be if crutches were being used on land, i.e. in the same order, and at the same distance apart. Four-point walking maintains the normal walking pattern, but the method taught must correspond to that on land. If bars are not available the hydrotherapist should support the patient at the pelvis. When normal supported walking has been established, free walking can be attempted, first forward and, later, backwards. Care must be taken to ensure that the affected heel is placed on the ground, and released only at the end of the step. Walking in any direction helps to mobilize the hip joint, and provides excellent muscle work for the hip abductors and extensors.

Stairs. Only the lower stairs should be attempted, and only after the patient has achieved even walking.

FINAL STAGES (12 to 16 weeks)

Entry by the stairs and the patient will be able to walk freely in the pool at this stage.

1. Half support side lying—on the affected side, adding float to affected leg—abduction of under leg.
2. Half support lying with knees bent and feet on a ring—hip and knee extension.
3. Half support lying—float at ankle—hip extension—add more floats.
4. Standing—circling affected leg—add float.
5. Side inclined standing affected leg uppermost with float— adduction of uppermost leg.

Swimming is to be encouraged since it exercises the whole of the lower limb, and improves, or enables the patient to achieve co-ordination with the other leg and the arms; in addition, the extensors of the back and the hip abductors are used strongly. Swimming is also very beneficial in giving the patient a sport which will enable him to maintain progress after he is discharged from hospital treatment.

In both breast stroke and back stroke the joint is abducted and laterally rotated, and therefore the muscles must be well developed and capable of guarding the joint before allowing these strokes to be performed. The crawl entails strong muscle work for the extensors of the hip and back; arm movements are taught in sitting, and the leg movements in prone lying; the two sets of movements should be combined to produce a stroke as soon as possible.

Ball games involving control of movement and balance can also be introduced. Exaggerated walking steps are another aid in help-ing the patient to gain the last few degrees of mobility, and achieve balance control. Walking in progressively shallower depths of water can be attempted at this stage, as the joint should be capable of bearing more weight. Similarly, the patient can practise walking up higher stairs.

The above scheme will be modified, of course, according to the capabilities of the patient, and the directions of the surgeon in charge. Some patients, for example, may be able to attempt swimming at an earlier stage; others may have swimming excluded from the treatment. Similarly, certain exercises may be unsuitable for elderly or weak patients, or the programme may need to include a few special exercises for the arm or shoulder if the joints are stiff or painful from crutch walking, or if the arms are weak and need strengthening for the task. A few selected exercises should be taught as home exercises.

SUGGESTED TREATMENT AFTER
ARTHRODESIS OF THE HIP

This operation is designed to give a pain-free, though stiffened joint. Following arthrodesis, it is imperative that the joints of the spine, knees and opposite hip are kept fully mobile, and that the muscles acting on these joints are well developed and strong; treatment is geared to this end.

If the fixation has not included the knee-joint full movements must be maintained, and the power of the quadriceps muscle increased to its maximum. Exercises for the opposite hip are carried out as previously described. Intensive mobilization will be necessary if the knee-joint on the affected side has been included in the fixation, and the exercises as for patellectomy (see below) are given.

Exercises (such as those detailed later for spinal conditions) are necessary to maintain or increase the mobility of the spine and improve the power of the abdominal and back extensor muscles. As the patient is usually young, energetic exercises can be given. If the feet are fixed under the pool rail, exercises moving the trunk on the pelvis can be incorporated in the support lying position. The patient can also be taught the butterfly stroke, which is especially useful as it can be performed without leg movements.

Walking, balance and postural re-education will be necessary, the trunk muscles being used to produce the movements of walking. Final rehabilitation follows the lines already described. Ball games involving trunk side flexion are invaluable in achieving balance control.

THE KNEE

With the exception of arthrodesis, surgery to the knee presents two problems: joint stiffness and quadriceps weakness. In almost every case the knee will have been extended during the period of immobilization, with the result that flexion has become limited. Pain and mechanical weakness before surgery may well have caused the quadriceps muscle to waste considerably, and the weak and unstable condition of the weight-bearing joint may be aggravated by disturbance of the extensor mechanisms during surgery and post-operative immobilization, producing even greater weakness. Treatment is therefore aimed at regaining quadriceps power and knee flexion. Normal flexion, though desirable, must not be gained at the expense of quadriceps power, however. Only when treatment has succeeded in restoring some measure of muscle strength, and the patient can again extend the knee, should active flexion be encouraged; if flexion is encouraged too soon, a quadriceps lag will result.

Synovectomy. Synovectomy of the knee may be treated in the pool approximately 2 weeks after surgery. This operation is often performed on a rheumatoid joint which may be deformed. Limitation of movement in other joints with associated muscle weakness may then be present, and would require treatment. Owing to deformity of the joint it may be impossible to obtain really full movement, but muscle strength should improve greatly.

Patellectomy. This operation is necessary for comminuted fracture or recurrent dislocation of the patella. The joint is immobilized for approximately 4 to 5 weeks post-operatively, after which time pool therapy may be started. As part of the stabilizing mechanism of the joint has been removed, complete muscle power must be regained to compensate for this. Many of these patients are young and strenuous exercises may be included in the final stages of treatment.

Menisectomy. Although pool therapy is not usually given after this operation, it may be ordered if the patient has difficulty in gaining full flexion or if the quadriceps are very weak. Mobilizing exercises and a full progression of strengthening exercises for the quadriceps are given on the lines already described.

Arthroplasty. This operation is performed on the traumatized or arthritic knee. Pool therapy is given approximately 3 to 4 weeks after surgery. Strengthening and mobilizing exercises are given as for the osteo-arthritic knee, and, at 4 to 5 weeks post-operatively, weight bearing in the pool can be allowed. Not more than 90° of flexion can be obtained, as further movement is impeded by the hinge prosthesis. Full weight bearing on land is delayed until 8 to 12 weeks after surgery; in the early stages of treatment, therefore, entry to the pool is by gantry apparatus.

Quadricepsplasty. Following injury to the lower third of the femur or to the knee-joint, quadricepsplasty may be necessary to regain flexion. After operation, fixation is in flexion and, though quadriceps exercises and active knee movements are started immediately, the patient is frequently left with a quadriceps lag.

Arthrodesis. This may be the method of choice to eliminate severe pain in a unilateral arthritis or fractured knee. The arthritic patient is especially prone to loss of movement in the hips, lumbar spine and ankle-joints, and mobilizing exercises are particularly important. Treatment in the pool begins approximately 2 months after operation.

In each of the above conditions re-education, following the treatment described for the hip, is necessary, in balance, posture, standing up, sitting down, walking and climbing stairs. The patient will also find swimming to be beneficial.

HYDROTHERAPY FOLLOWING SURGERY OF THE UPPER LIMB

THE SHOULDER

The commonest reasons for surgery at the shoulder are recurrent dislocation, fracture and rheumatoid arthritis.

Recurrent dislocation. The two most widely employed techniques are those described by Bankart and Putti-Platt. In every case the operation is designed to secure the head of the humerus and to approximate its articular surface with the glenoid cavity. Fixation is usually for 3 to 6 weeks with the arm by the side, the elbow bent and the hand resting on the opposite shoulder. Mobilization in the pool is started as soon as possible after the fixation is removed. Full shoulder movement should be gained eventually, with the exception of some degrees of lateral rotation; after the Putti-Platt operation the last degree of true abduction may also be lost.

Axillary nerve damage and weakness or even paralysis of the deltoid muscle may result from a dislocated shoulder. Suitable exercises are outlined in Chapter 8.

In the early stages of treatment, exercises for all movements are to be encouraged, with buoyancy assisting. Re-education should be started with the patient in the sitting position, so that the hydrotherapist can see every direction of movement and can control the tendency for scapulo-humeral rhythm to be reversed. As more mobility is gained, exercises can be given, using floats or buoyancy as a resistance. Modified facilitation techniques can be introduced with the patient in the float support lying position. For example, the arm can be elevated through abduction and lateral rotation, returning by adduction and medial rotation; the movement finishes with the hand at the mid-line of the trunk. Swimming, too, is excellent for gaining full mobility and should be encouraged at the earliest opportunity. Correction of posture should be continued throughout treatment.

Arthroplasty. This may be necessary owing to a fracture-dislocation of the head of the humerus or for rheumatoid arthritis of the shoulder joint. A Neer's type prothesis may be used. Exercises are begun as soon as the sutures are removed, usually 2 to 3 weeks after operation. Mobilizing exercises are begun immediately, the programme of treatment being similar to that for other shoulder conditions. Full-range shoulder movements are seldom regained, although adequate functional movement can be expected.

Similarly, dislocation of the acromioclavicular or sternoclavicular joints may require surgical intervention, and after a specified period of fixation, re-education of shoulder movements and posture will be necessary.

THE ELBOW

Excision arthroplasty (removal of the head of the radius). Arthroplasty of the elbow may be required after a compound fracture or fracture dislocation. While this is not usually treated in the pool in the early stages, hydrotherapy may be the selected method of starting exercise. Mobilization begins some 10 days to 2 weeks after surgery, with flexion and extension and pronation and supination exercises for the elbow. These movements should be encouraged gently, and on no account must they be forced. The emphasis is on increasing muscle strength, particularly of the triceps and biceps. Instability of the joint is likely to follow arthroplasty, unless adequate muscle control is regained. Movements for the shoulder-joint must be encouraged as the patient will otherwise tend to hold his arm still and to the side. Elbow movements are started in the sitting position.

EARLY STAGE

All movements of the elbow will be weak, and limited:
1. Reach sitting with palms downwards—elbow bending and stretching.
2. Sitting—elbow bending and stretching.
3. Sitting with elbows flexed and palms upwards—pronation and supination.

LATER STAGES

Exercise (1) is progressed by placing the forearm in the midposition with the thumb pointing upwards; the movement then meets more resistance from the water. As the movement becomes stronger, the speed of performance can be increased, or the patient can hold a float or bat.

Resisted elbow extension can be performed from the bend-sitting position, and combined elbow and shoulder movements can be encouraged. The arm movements of breast stroke, which involve flexion and extension, pronation and supination of the elbow, can be taught in sitting, and later performed with the patient holding floats to increase resistance. Elbow and shoulder extension can be achieved by stretching the arm from the across bend position, while both flexion and extension can be encouraged by pushing balls through the water.

FINAL STAGES

Strenuous exercises involving pushing and pulling can now be introduced to gain full muscle power and the final degrees of movement:
1. Grasp standing between parallel bars with elbows semiflexed—elbow straightening to lift body off pool floor.
2. Stretch grasp prone lying—elbow flexion and extension.

Swimming, too, is beneficial as it necessitates the arms taking the weight of the body through the water, and thus demands hard muscle work from the biceps and triceps.

THE SPINE

Two surgical procedures commonly performed on the spine are laminectomy and spinal fusion. Patients having undergone these operations can be treated successfully by hydrotherapy as soon as movement can be encouraged.

Laminectomy. Laminectomy may be carried out after fracture or fracture dislocation of the vertebrae or, more commonly, for a prolapsed intervertebral disc. Disc protrusion usually occurs in the lumbar region, and in 80 per cent of cases, the sciatic nerve is involved, with referred pain in the buttocks or legs. Gross muscle weakness of the back, glutei and legs may result from inactivity and sciatic pain, and in turn, muscle weakness can cause limping or awkward gait. Postural defects such as lumbar scoliosis may be present. Paraplegia may also result from a fracture of the spine, and suitable treatment is outlined in Chapter 8.

Pool therapy begins 2 to 4 weeks after operation according to the surgeon's directions. Weight bearing is allowed at about the same time. Post-operative treatment includes back and leg exercises, correction of posture and instruction in balance, walking and swimming.

Two schools of thought govern the selection of exercises. Some authorities affirm that only back extension exercises should be taught post-operatively, and that flexion of the spine, if allowed at all, need not be encouraged. Others, however, insist that flexion should be encouraged to prevent fibrous tissue from forming round the intervertebral foramen and interfering with the nerve roots. Rotation and trunk side flexion is allowed whichever treatment is chosen.

The following is a guide to treatment for the back, following laminectomy:

EARLY STAGES (2 to 4 weeks after operation)

Exercises are chosen to strengthen all affected and weak muscles, and to increase or maintain the range of movement in the vertebral and hip joints. The treatment should be given in fixed or semi-fixed positions, with buoyancy eliminated or used to assist movements. Quadriceps exercises are necessary, to gain control and muscle power for walking and to prepare for instruction on correct lifting. The patient should be taught to correct his pelvic tilt and posture.

Throughout the following *spinal flexion is avoided:*

1. Support prone lying on inclined plinth—alternate hip extension.
2. Heave grasp float support lying—trunk side flexion by moving legs.
3. Float support side lying—back extension.
4. Float support lying—correction of posture.
5. Float support lying—shoulder retraction.
6. Float support lying—legs parting and closing.
7. Reach grasp standing—re-education of walking.

With *spinal flexion allowed*, the following exercises may be added:

1. Support lying on inclined plinth—alternate straight leg raising.
2. Reach grasp standing—alternate hip flexion.
3. Support side lying—flexion of hips and knees on to chest and extension.

LATER STAGES (4 to 6 weeks)

Muscle power will have increased, so that more strenuous exercises can be introduced against the resistance of buoyancy:

With *spinal flexion avoided:*

1. Half support lying—hip extension.
2. Half support lying—swinging one leg over opposite leg, returning to start position.
3. Half float support lying, feet under rail—trunk side flexion.
4. Half support lying—leg movements of back crawl.
5. Reach grasp standing—one hip and knee flexed to 90°, float round ankle, knee and hip extension.
6. Float support lying with feet under rail—float in hands—extend the arms into the water.
7. Standing—correction of posture.
8. Float lying—back extension patterns using arms.

With *spinal flexion allowed*, exercises (2), (3), (4), (5) as above, and:

1. Half support prone lying—hip and knee flexion to bring knees under plinth followed by extension. Add floats.
2. Half support prone lying—leg movements of crawl and breast stroke.
3. Float support lying—flexion and extension patterns.

FINAL STAGES (5 to 10 weeks)

Strong resisted exercises may now be introduced and swimming encouraged. All strokes provide good work for the trunk muscles and help to increase power; back stroke and crawl are particularly useful for extension while breast stroke and butterfly may be included as exercises involving flexion. Trunk rotation is achieved in the arm movements of crawl and in the flexion-extension-rotation patterns. Ball games involving rotation and balance may be included in the table of exercises. Progression through each stage should be made as quickly as the patient's capabilities will allow.

Spinal fusion. Treatment of patients following a spinal fusion follows the extension method previously described but with two differences. Firstly, pool therapy will begin later than after laminectomy; and secondly flexion will be delayed until the final stages of treatment.

Spinal fusion with screw fixation is treated approximately 8 to 10 weeks after operation. Back extension exercises, re-education in walking and correction of posture are given with more difficult exercises introduced gradually. At 16 to 18 weeks gentle flexion may be started if the X-rays show no contra-indications. Gradually the range is increased, function being restored to normal after about six months.

Following an 'H graft' hydrotherapy begins at 24 weeks. Again the initial emphasis is on extension, flexion being introduced gradually at a much later stage. Final recovery may take up to a year.

CHRONIC DISABILITIES

Some chronic orthopaedic conditions may be treated in the pool to relieve pain or to maintain or increase joint movement and muscle strength.

9

Paget's disease. This disease is characterized by absorption of calcium from the bones, accompanied by new soft bone formation, with weakness and deformity of the affected bones, usually the pelvic girdle, spine, femur and clavicle. Pool therapy is particularly beneficial when the weight-bearing bones are affected.

CONDITIONS PRODUCING BACK PAIN

Spondylolithesis and spondylolisis. Pain is usually felt in the lumbar region and in the legs. Back extension exercises and general leg exercises are given. Correction of posture and instruction in walking may be necessary.

Disc protrusion. The conservative treatment of disc protrusions includes a period of rest followed by exercises. Pool therapy may begin 2 to 6 weeks after the onset of pain but longer rest may be necessary if root signs are present. Strengthening exercises for the back and general leg exercises are given. In the final stages of rehabilitation controlled flexion exercises may be ordered by some surgeons. The exercises given will be progressed on similar lines to those suggested following laminectomy.

Spondylosis. General back mobilizing exercises may be given for this condition but as rotation is painful in the early stages this should be avoided initially. Extension or flexion exercises may be given depending on the doctor's wishes.

Strains or partial or complete rupture of the ligaments of the back. Mobilizing and strengthening exercises are given within the limits of pain, progressing to full-range movements as the pain is alleviated. All spinal movements can be attempted.

Postural defects (without bony changes). For all postural defects the tables of exercises described in the section on back surgery are suitable. Arm exercises should be included in the treatment, while swimming is of great benefit for these conditions. Correction of posture and pelvic tilt in lying, sitting and standing is necessary.

    1. Kyphosis. Extension, side flexion and rotation exercises are given. The crawl and back crawl swimming strokes are to be encouraged for extension of the hips and spine, while underwater swimming may be used to help increase the patient's vital capacity.

    2. Scoliosis. General exercises are given, and all the swimming strokes can be attempted. If the scoliosis has followed surgery for

a lung condition, underwater swimming may be introduced to improve the patient's vital capacity.

3. Flat back. General exercises may be given, and any of the swimming strokes taught.

SOFT TISSUE INJURIES

Synovitis and bursitis. These conditions may be treated in the pool in the subacute or chronic stages. Movement becomes less inhibited as pain is relieved and muscle spasm reduced, and exercises to increase muscle power and range of movement are then given.

Synovitis or bursitis of the knee is relatively common, and when chronic, quadriceps insufficiency and joint instability will be apparent. Extension exercises may improve the condition.

Arm exercises, performed with gravity and buoyancy eliminated, may be beneficial for a chronic subacromial bursitis. Abduction with lateral rotation to elevation may be given in the support lying position, to avoid movement against gravity, through the 'painful arc'.

Ruptured ligaments. Partially ruptured ligaments are immobilized until healing is complete, but if the rupture is complete, suturing becomes necessary. Following rupture of the medial or lateral ligaments of the knee-joint, 6 to 8 weeks should elapse before mobilization begins. After a cruciate rupture, however, mobilization can be started earlier, at approximately 3 to 4 weeks. Suitable exercises are outlined in the section on osteo-arthritis of the knees.

FRACTURES

FRACTURES OF THE FEMUR IN THE ELDERLY

Fractured neck (intracapsular). Whether the fracture is impacted or displaced, fixation is usually by insertion of a Smith–Petersen pin, unless the femur is osteoporotic when an Austin Moore type prosthesis is used instead. Mobilization in the pool can begin 10 to 14 days after injury. Great care should be taken with the elderly patient, and the hydrotherapist must take time to reassure him and explain the treatment to be given. Initially, exercises are given for the hip and knee, using buoyancy to assist the movement, or with buoyancy supporting the moving part; buoyancy as resistance is added as soon as possible. All movements of the hip-joint can be carried out, with the exception of lateral rotation. Emphasis is on strengthening the abductors and extensors of the hip and regaining functional movement. Re-education in weight transference, balance and walking should be started at the earliest opportunity and any limping corrected. Instruction in stair-climbing will also be necessary. By 6 to 8 weeks all movements should have been regained adequately, including lateral rotation; the patient will then be virtually independent.

Trochanteric fracture (*extracapsular*). Fixation is usually by inserting a nail plate. Pool therapy is started 10 to 14 days after injury with graduated exercises for the hip and knee and walking being taught from the first attendance. Lateral rotation is restricted until 3 or 4 weeks after operation.

FRACTURES OF THE FEMUR IN THE YOUNG

Conservative treatment may be recommended for an undisplaced impacted fracture.

Fractured neck (*intracapsular*). Pool treatment is started approximately 3 to 4 weeks after injury, and following a period in traction. Full weight-bearing on land must be delayed until 10 to 12 weeks after injury, but walking in water can be introduced at 4 to 5 weeks. Emphasis should be laid on mobilizing the hip-joint, and strengthening the muscles acting upon it. Quadriceps power also has to be improved, and the knee—stiffened through traction—must be mobilized. Swimming is introduced as soon as the patient can manage this, and re-education of walking, posture, balance and climbing stairs carried out. Progression is quicker than in surgical cases and full rehabilitation should be achieved in 3 to 4 months.

Trochanteric fracture (*extracapsular*). Conservative treatment necessitates 10 to 12 weeks on traction until the fracture is united; pool therapy is then begun. Mobilization of the hip and knee, and strengthening of the muscles acting on these joints, are the chief aims of treatment in the early stages, although exercises for the lumbar spine should also be included. When partial weight-bearing is allowed on land, the patient can be taught to walk in the pool, and is encouraged to swim. Postural correction must be given throughout treatment. Progression will be slower than after a fractured neck, full rehabilitation taking 5 to 8 months.

FRACTURES OF THE SHAFT

Conservative treatment. Pool therapy is begun 12 to 16 weeks after injury. Mobilization of the hip, knee and spine will be necessary, and strengthening of all the muscles acting on these joints essential. Knee movements will be very limited, and the quadriceps muscles weak after the long period in continuous traction. Walking can begin early in treatment, and more vigorous exercises introduced as progress is made. In the later stages of therapy resisted leg exercises using floats and flippers will prove beneficial; swimming should be encouraged. These patients are usually young and later exercise can be vigorous. Full rehabilitation may take up to a year.

Surgical treatment. Internal fixation by intra-medullary nail may be used if satisfactory reduction cannot be achieved by conservative measures. Pool therapy is started 4 to 6 weeks after operation, with mobilizing and strengthening exercises as above. Walking should be delayed until 6 to 8 weeks after operation.

FRACTURES AROUND THE KNEE-JOINT

Such fractures inevitably lead to limitation of movement and weakness of the quadriceps muscles. When the limb is immobilized in a full-length plaster, hydrotherapy is delayed for some weeks.

The patient first enters the pool by hoist, and is given active exercises for the knee. Emphasis is put upon acquiring full extension and good quadriceps power. Full flexion must not be gained at the expense of full extension, as a quadriceps lag and instability of the joint would result. Walking can begin at an early stage, and hip movements should be included in the exercise programme; exercises to improve balance and posture must be given. Later, the patient can be taught to swim and to walk up and down stairs.

Mobilizing and strengthening exercises for the knee are the same as for osteo-arthritis. If the joint remains stiff, manipulative treatment may be given, after which vigorous exercises must produce the same range of movement as under anaesthetic.

Supracondylar and condylar fractures. Pool therapy is started approximately 6 to 7 weeks after injury. With these fractures injury to the lateral popliteal nerve may occur, producing dropped foot, for which re-education is the same as for other peripheral nerve injuries. A toe-raising device, made from tape and elastic with Velcro fastening may be used to assist walking in the pool.

Fractured patella. Depending on the severity of fracture, mobilization can begin from the third day to the third week after injury, when the emphasis must be on gaining good quadriceps contraction; knee movements should be encouraged gradually.

Following suture or pinning of an avulsion fracture of the patella, pool exercises can be given to mobilize the knee and strengthen the quadriceps once the plaster has been removed (usually 3 to 4 weeks after operation).

Avulsion of the tibial spine. Pool therapy is begun about 6 weeks after surgery.

FRACTURED SHAFTS OF TIBIA AND FIBULA

Mobilization is allowed approximately 12 to 16 weeks after injury. Because the period of fixation is so long, gross limitation of movement in the knee- and ankle-joints with weakness of the quadriceps hamstrings, calf and anterior tibial muscles are usual. Exercises for all affected joints and muscles must be given. Instruction in walking, balance and posture can be given from the start of treatment with swimming and stair-climbing being introduced as the patient progresses.

FRACTURE AND FRACTURE DISLOCATION OF THE ANKLE

These fractures are seldom treated in the pool unless the patient also has other conditions or fractures which are to be treated by the hydrotherapist. Mobilization is then begun 3 to 12 weeks after injury, depending on the severity of the fracture and the period of fixation. Ankle movements and general leg exercises should be given, together with instruction in balance, walking and posture.

FRACTURES AROUND THE SHOULDER JOINT

Limitation of movement and muscle weakness are the chief characteristics of virtually all fractures around the shoulder joint. In the early stages there may also be oedema and haematoma. Many patients sustaining such injuries are elderly, and disinclined to move the affected arm, holding it rigidly by the side. As soon as mobilization is allowed active exercises must be performed, to regain movement and restore strength. It is also necessary to correct reversed humero-scapular rhythm, so that trick movements do not develop. Elbow and hand exercises should be included in the treatment, especially if swelling is present. In the later stages, provided that it is suitable for the patient, swimming can be introduced, the arm movements of both breast stroke and crawl being excellent for mobilizing the stiff shoulder.

FRACTURED NECK OF HUMERUS

With an *impacted* fracture, pool therapy can begin 2 to 3 days after injury, with active assisted shoulder exercises using buoyancy, and the patient either lying or sitting. As the fracture is so recent oedema and bruising will be present making movement acutely painful. Reassurance and encouragement should be given and care taken to prevent unguarded movements. The warmth of the water relieves pain, and relaxation of the shoulder muscles may be gained by gentle kneading under the water. Active movements are progressed as quickly as possible, and swimming introduced, if suitable. Full rehabilitation should be achieved in 6 to 8 weeks.

With an *unimpacted* fracture, shoulder movements can be started 3 weeks from injury. Rehabilitation takes slightly longer than with an impacted fracture, owing to a greater degree of joint stiffness. Initial movements are not so painful, however.

A young patient with a *displaced unimpacted fracture* may not begin pool therapy for 6 to 7 weeks. Limitation of movement in the elbow-joint will accompany the restricted movement of the shoulder, and mobilizing and strengthening exercises will be necessary for both joints.

The axillary nerve may be involved in any of the above fractures, incurring inability to abduct the arm, and weakness of lateral rotation. The necessary re-education is as for other peripheral nerve injuries.

Fracture of the greater tuberosity. Pool therapy is started about 2 weeks after injury, active shoulder exercises being given to regain mobility and strength. An associated supraspinatus syndrome may require treatment.

FRACTURED SHAFT OF HUMERUS

Treatment follows a relatively long period of immobilization, beginning 6 to 8 weeks after injury, the whole limb being included in the treatment. If fixation has involved the forearm, limitation of the elbow movements will be evident, in addition to stiffness of the shoulder. Exercises to restore the mobility of the forearm and the strength of the biceps and triceps, will therefore be necessary.

Active shoulder exercises should be progressed rapidly, and resisted movements and swimming introduced as soon as the patient is able to tackle them. Functional recovery should be complete in 3 to 4 months.

If the radial nerve has been involved, a 'dropped' wrist may result, and must be treated.

Mobilization and rehabilitation is quicker when the shaft is fixed internally with an intramedullary nail, than when a conservative treatment is adopted.

FRACTURES OF THE SPINE

Conservative treatment of fractures of the spine involves a period of rest, and later, exercises to increase joint mobility and muscle power. Emphasis is on gaining extension of the spine and increasing the power of the extensor muscles. Flexion is allowed in the later stages of treatment. Swimming can be encouraged from the beginning, however, as a means of providing strong work for the extensor muscles. Suitable extension exercises are outlined in the section on back surgery.

Compression fracture of the vertebral bodies. Pool exercises will begin 4 to 12 weeks after injury depending on the severity of the fracture. The exercises, as above, are progressed quickly, and recovery should be in 3 to 6 months.

Fracture dislocation of the spine. If the spinal cord has escaped injury, reduction and fixation is attempted by insertion of a metal plate. Several weeks after injury, back extension exercises and leg exercises may be taught. Re-education of walking, balance and posture will be necessary. Partial or complete recovery takes several months.

If the cord has been severed completely, treatment is as for a paraplegia.

Fracture of transverse processes. Exercises may be given 2 weeks after injury and full recovery should be gained in a few weeks.

DISLOCATIONS

The hip. Dislocation of the hip is unusual. Following reduction and a long period of fixation, limitation of movement and muscle weakness is inevitable. Mobilizing exercises and exercises to strengthen the hip muscles are given on similar lines to those described under hip surgery.

The knee. If the ligaments of the knee are ruptured or stretched violently the tibia can be displaced in any direction on the femur, thereby dislocating the knee-joint. Following reduction and fixation pool therapy is started at 8 to 10 weeks after injury, limitation of movement and weakness of the quadriceps muscles demanding mobilizing and strengthening exercises. The programme of treatment follows that outlined in the section on osteo-arthritis of the knee. Peripheral nerves around the joint may also be injured, necessitating further treatment.

The shoulder. Once the dislocation has been reduced, the shoulder can be mobilized, beginning within the first few days with the elderly patient but often delayed for 3 weeks with the young patient. In the early stages of treatment careful watch should be kept for the onset of an axillary nerve lesion. The elderly patient often has considerable pain and bruising and for these patients the pool is a particularly useful method of treatment. All shoulder movements can be given but some authorities prefer lateral rotation to be delayed for a week. In the early stages it is only given with the arm by the side. All movements are gradually progressed to full range and given against the resistance of buoyancy. Swimming is included for any patient who is capable of it. With the younger patient all movements may be given from the beginning.

The elbow. Dislocation of this joint is unlikely to be treated in the pool unless associated with a fracture around the elbow joint.

10

Children in Water

CHILDREN who are handicapped need not be denied the delight of movement. Physical activity on land may be hard for such children, but in the water they come into their own. Most children enjoy the water and want to learn to swim, and the sense of achievement when they master the art is enormous. They gain in confidence, their self-respect is enhanced and they acquire a social benefit, for in the water they can compete with their normal counterparts. Handicapped children, like others, benefit from incentives to improve their stamina and technique; therefore, the effects are both psychological and physical.

A child must experience active movement if he is to develop, and lack of physical experience may well be a major factor in the slow development of the handicapped child. Activity in the water is a means of widening his experience, although hydrotherapy, in its strictly accepted sense of being purely remedial, is not of great value when taking children into the water. If a child is asked whether he would like to play about in the water he would most probably reply, 'Yes'; therefore any programme of exercise should be hidden by playing. This can be given a positive aspect if the programme is designed to include the teaching of swimming with the remedial exercises.

A definite approach now emerges, as few children, however timorous, can resist joining in with those happily at play. It is essential that the child is mentally happy in the water as well as being physically adjusted, so that the most beneficial atmosphere can be created. This means that he must be completely balanced in an element which is naturally strange to him. The mental adjustment cannot be obtained by assurance on the part of the hydrotherapist that, 'Everything will be alright'. It can only come from within the child, whose sense of balance in the water must be developed in such a manner as to give him self-assurance.

The understanding of the element of water, and the continual adjustment to its feel, its turbulence, its buoyancy and its weight—especially where these may affect the body balance—are vitally important, and together with the technique of breathing control both in and under the water, should be the background to all pool activities. Correct breathing control should be taught continually; likewise the ability to recover to a safe breathing position.

There are two extremes of posture—being stretched out full length and being doubled up as a ball. The upright position, standing on a relatively small area, is disturbed easily and rotates about its longitudinal axis but the rolled up position provides stable balance and considerable effort is required to change the position of the body. Therefore, all early activities and exercises should be carried out in shapes that tend to be 'balled up' (Fig. 49). As the child develops balance and control these shapes should be 'unrolled' to become longer, thus requiring a greater degree of control. These two positions are described as 'ball' and 'stick'.

As creatures of land, with all the subconscious patterns of land

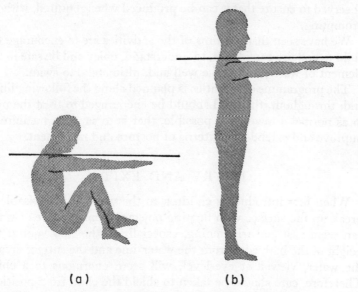

(a) (b)

Fig. 49. (a) 'Ball'; (b) 'stick' or upright

living, many are apprehensive and tense in the water, and the handicapped child is likely to have other and specific inhibitions which arise as a result of his physical disability. He may suffer, for example, from a very acute fear of falling, difficulty of communication, inability to move readily or at will, inability to control sporadic or unwanted movement, poor or badly controlled respiration, lack of comprehension and asymmetry in shape and density.

In all programmes of activity the fullest range of sensation and movement should be used, change of pace, change of position, change of atmosphere from seriousness to laughter. Such phrases as 'lying in bed', 'head on the pillow', 'rolling over', 'sitting in your chair' are associated with land habits and safety. Negative expressions such as 'sinking', 'drowning', 'holding the breath', 'shutting the eyes' should *never* be used.

Exercises, activities and games should be constructed on the following lines: a primary game in which the child is shown and, if necessary, assisted in the creation of a movement or a shape; a follow-up activity requiring the child to create the movement or shape against the effect and weight of moving water; and, finally, an oblique activity which may suggest a different objective to the child but still contains the primary activity—the movement is then observed to ensure that it can be produced when required, without prompting.

We have seen that the aims of the activities are to encourage the child to acquire confidence, to understand, enjoy and be safe in the element of water, to breathe well and, ultimately, to swim.

The programme of activities is planned along the following lines, and, throughout, the child should be encouraged to treat the pool in as normal a manner as possible, that is to say as a medium to improve and extend his patterns of posture and movement.

ENTRY AND EXIT

When first introducing children to the water it is advisable to break up the surface with floating objects, as an expanse of water can seem vast and frightening, especially to the very young: the height of the bath edge from the water-line and the surface area of the water, viewed at eye-level, will seem enormous to a child. Therefore, care should be taken to shield the child from positions that accentuate height and distance. For instance, short-distance focal points can be achieved by working across the shortest distance of the pool, by facing into a corner, or by allowing interesting objects to float on the water within sight of the child.

A method of entry and exit over the side of the bath, that the child can manage for himself in due course, is advisable for he may not always swim in a pool where steps or a ramp and help are available to get him in and out of the water.

Once in the water the hydrotherapist should remember always to adopt a position which enables the child to see and communicate without disturbing his balance unnecessarily. If the therapist is standing in the water, her height above the child will cause him to tilt his head back to see her, and in so doing his feet will swing forward and upwards. To achieve rapport with the child it is vital that he has a feeling of closeness and can see the hydrotherapist at his own eye-level and can also converse comfortably with her. This is especially necessary with children who are partially deaf as poor acoustics are usual in the pool.

When working behind the child the hydrotherapist should stand where any slight turn by the child gives him a view of the hydrotherapist's face. Likewise, she should always be in such a position that her lips are close to the child's ears so that her instruction can be given in a clear and quiet manner.

BREATHING CONTROL

Holding the breath is a major factor in the creation of tension within the body; therefore, the child must be told to blow when the water is near his face. The effect of blowing tends to bring the head forward in an aggressive action, in contrast to the loss of head control that follows the withdrawal or flinching action of the head when water is splashed on the face.

Before embarking on any other activity it is advisable to ensure that the child has blown bubbles and has also wet his face. The latter can be achieved by playing splashing games or by 'washing' his own face. Breathing is continually combined with other activities to ensure that the child is developing a natural rhythm essential to anyone involved in activity in water.

SAFETY AND RECOVERY

The child must be taught how to use his head to control the position of his body, so that, at all times, he can regain a safe breathing position. Such control can be achieved by one of the two movements described below, or by a combination of both.

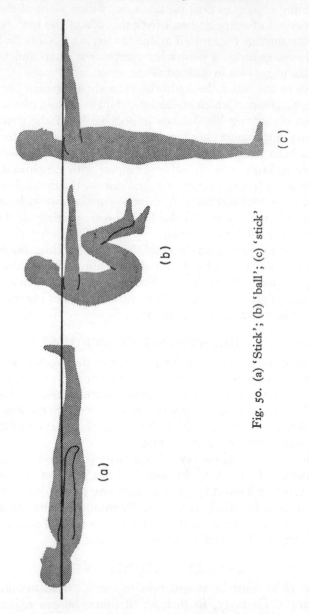

Fig. 50. (a) 'Stick'; (b) 'ball'; (c) 'stick'

The first movement, from lying on the back to standing, is achieved by bringing the body into a 'balled-up' position and by forcing the head forward, causing the body to rotate forward. When the head is vertical the body is unrolled into the standing position. When lying, the child must be able to control any axial rotation of his body which can occur either as a result of the asymmetry due to his handicap or because the movement of either the water or his body disturbs his position.

REMEDIAL EXERCISES

Many of these can be incorporated in other activities, specific treatment varies according to need.

ACTIVITIES

The simple skills of standing, walking, jumping—both forwards and backwards—and turning in the water must be acquired as a basis for independence, and to prepare the child for swimming. All activities should begin with the stable, 'ball' position. As control improves the child can be encouraged to unroll his body into the 'stick' position to achieve more finely-balanced movements.

If the body is formed into a ball, and a position adopted on the floor of the bath, the child will come to the surface quickly. This can be conveyed to children in games demanding that they sit on the floor and stay there; they will find this impossible as the water pushes them up. However, before any activity below the surface is undertaken adequate breathing control must be established.

Care should be taken with children suffering from cerebral palsy, especially in the early stages, to avoid the effects of extensor thrust of the head and neck under the water. In addition, before carrying out underwater activity a check should be made for any similar movement that could cause the mouth to be opened involuntarily.

Floatation equipment. The use of floating equipment—except when a specific effect is required in remedial exercises—is highly undesirable, and in some cases dangerous. Each handicapped person has a balance problem peculiar to himself, the effect of which can be altered completely or even reversed. Thus extreme care must be used in adjusting floatation equipment to ensure that the required balance position is maintained under any circumstance.

The use of floatation equipment obviates one of the greatest advantages of working in the water, that of developing a finer degree of balance control.

HOLDS

The way in which the child is held in the water can affect the development of balance. The main object must always be to give the child the maximum feel of his own balanced position with the minimum of support. Whatever his body position he should be held near or opposite to his centre of buoyancy approximately the lower end of the sternum. Although in the early stages the child may grip the hydrotherapist, this should be reduced eventually to a light hold, as gripping induces tension and destroys the sense of balance. In the facing position, the child's hands should be placed on the therapist's in such a manner that the extended hands are at the level of the lower end of the sternum. A finger-tip support should be given at the same level when the child has his back to the hydrotherapist, or is lying on his back.

There is no limit to the games and activities that can be devised, and it is hoped that the above will serve as a basis upon which to work. Objectives can be achieved through recreation but should not be lost in the enjoyment of water activity. Greater benefit can sometimes be derived from group treatment, and often the child enjoys such activity and benefits from the companionship it offers.

Whatever the handicap the aims of the programme remain the same, and activity in the water has its place in the overall development and pattern of the child's life.

EXAMPLES OF GAMES

1. A game performed in the upright 'stick' position, and requiring head control can be developed in the following manner:

Primary activity

Purpose: head control.

Appreciation: water has weight.

Formation: a circle is formed, swimmer and hydrotherapist alternately, all holding hands and facing inwards.

Instruction: to walk round sideways taking a step and bringing the other foot to it, lean and push against the water, when the water comes near your face—blow.

The points to watch are that the head is inclined in the direction the circle is moving, and that it is maintained in such a position that the feet remain in contact with the floor of the bath and do not rise forwards or backwards, and that the feet do not cross.

Follow-up activity

The purpose and formation remain the same but appreciation is increased in that when the swimmer feels the weight of water moving against him, he must push.

Instruction: to walk sideways, clockwise, when the word change is given, alter direction to anticlockwise.

Once the circle is moving well and the water is turbulent the direction 'change' is given to ensure that the swimmer works with his head and trunk to move in the reverse direction.

Oblique activity

The purpose, appreciation and formation are the same again.

Instruction: to walk round sideways stepping in the rhythm of a song, for example, 'There was a crooked man who walked a crooked mile.' The singing must continue even when the direction is changed.

The point to watch here is that head control is subconsciously exerted and the swimmer is given plenty to remember to ensure that the reaction is automatic.

2. A game using the 'ball' position:

Primary activity

Purpose: head control and body balance.

Appreciation: effect of the movement of the head on the body position in the water.

Formation: a circle is formed, alternately swimmer and hydro-therapist holding hands and facing inwards.

Instruction: swimmers bend your knees up towards your chests and slowly move your heads forwards and backwards.

Assistance is given to the swimmer, by the hydrotherapists moving their arms forwards and backwards slightly. It is important that the head control forwards and backwards is such that the 'balled-up' body does not swing too far.

Follow-up activity

The purpose, appreciation and formation remain the same.
Instruction: add to the previous instruction to sing a song—for
example, Frère Jacques—and swing to its rhythm.

It is important to watch for automatic control by the head of the
body swing, and that 'blowing' occurs when the face is near the
water on the forward movement.

Oblique activity

This follows the pattern of the above but can be progressed so
that the body is gradually unrolled, a larger swing occurring but
the head still controlling the body so that no sudden upthrust of
the legs occurs.

3. Underwater activity:

With the use of objects that will sink slowly the swimmer can
begin to reach for them close to the surface, blowing when the
water is near his face and gradually going deeper and deeper. He
will have to keep his eyes open to see the object, important in all
underwater activity, and also learn good breathing control and
how to work down against the buoyancy of the water.

Index

Figures printed in bold type indicate a definition or main description

Accidents, 42, 44, 45
Activities, children, 117, 118, 119, 120
    functional, 25, 64, 67, 71, 77, 79, 80, 84, 85, 90, 91
    recreational, 25, 48, 64, 67, 83
    underwater, 120
Acute anterior poliomyelitis, 72, **82**
Adhesion, 14
Advantages, 24
Amputations, 92
Ankylosing spondylitis, **67**
Archimedes' principle, **6**
Arthrodesis, 93, 96, 98
Arthroplasty, 92, 97, 99
Artificial respiration, 45
Assisted movement, *see* Movement
Ataxia, cerebellar, 74
    sensory, 74
Axonotomesis, 84

Back stroke, 67, 68, 95
Balance, 26, 78, 90, 101, 108, 113, 118, 119
    re-education, 89, 91, 93, 98, 110
Bay, 51
Blood pressure, 22, 23, 60, 75
    supply, 21, 22, 24, 74
Breast stroke, 67, 68, 83, 95, 100
Breathing control, 113, **115**, 120
Breathing exercises, *see* Exercises
Buoyancy, 4, 6, **8**, 9, 10, 11, 12, 24, 25, 29, 30, 32, 33, 40, 43, 50, 72, 85, 88, 113
    centre of, **9**, 10
    moment of, **9**, 10

Burns, 44
Bursitis, 105
Butterfly stroke, 96

Calorifier, 53
Cardiovascular disorders, 59
Centre of buoyancy, *see* Buoyancy
Centre of gravity, *see* Gravity
Cerebral accident, 75
Cerebral palsy, 58, 117
Cerebral thrombosis, 60
Children, 112
Chill, 23, 28
Chlorination, 25, 45, 52, 78
Chlorous, 45, 46
Cohesion, **14**, 15
Coordination, 26, 73, 82, 88, 90, 91
Contra-indications, 26, 58, **59**
Contractures, 73, 79, 82, 84
Crawl, 83, 95, 104
    back, 79, 104
    front, 64, 104
Crutches, 8, 28, 42, 55

Dangers, 42, 43
Deformity, 61, 73, 85, 88, 90, 91
    flexion, 65, 68
Density, 4, 5, 7, 8, 12
    relative, 5
Depth of pool, *see* Pool
Dermatitis, 26
Disadvantages of pool therapy, 24, 25
Disc protrusion, 104
Dislocations, 92
    elbow, 111

Dislocations—*cont.*
  hip, 110
  knee, 111
  recurrent, 98
  shoulder, 98, 111
Drowning, 45
Dyne, 4, **5**

Eddies, 17, 18
Effects, therapeutic, **24**, 25, 40
  untoward, **23**, 27
Epilepsy, 59
Examination of patient, **26**
Exercise, graduated, 61, 62, 76
  progression, 19, 24, 29, 85, 90
Exercises, arm, 80
  back, 62, 101, 103, 104, 110
  breathing, 75
  extensor pattern arm, 39, 40
  extensor pattern leg, 38, 39
  hip, 93, 105
  knee, 93, 105
  leg, 80, 101
  mobilizing, 99
  trunk, 78, 80

Fatigue, 23, 24, 53
Fixation, 25, 34, 38
Flaccidity, 58, 72, 75
Floats, 11, 24, 29, 33, 38, **55**, 62
Fluid loss, 23, 27
Foot-bath, 46, 52
Force, 15
  moment of, **9**, 10, 11
Fractures, 58, 92, **105**
  ankle, 108
  around knee, 107
    shoulder, 108
  femur, 105
    supracondylar, 107
  humerus, 109
  patella, 108
  tibia and fibula, 108
Fracture dislocation, of the ankle, 108
  of the spine, 110

Gait, 90

Games, 77, 83, 114, 118, 119, 120
  ball, 80, 95, 96
Gantry, *see* Hoist,
Gases, 4
Gravity, 4, 8, 12
  centre of, 8, 9
  specific, 4, **5**, 6, 8

Handrail, 43, 44, **52**, 57
Headrest, **55**
Heart rate, 22
Heat gain, 21
  loss, 21, 23
Hemiplegia, 58, 72, **75**
Hoist, **54**
Hold-relax technique, 40, 41, 90
Hubbard tank, **51**
Humidity, 53
Hydrostatic pressure, 4, **9**
Hypertension, 60
Hypotension, 60

Ice, 5, 45
Incontinence, 59, 77, 79
Incoordination, 74, 89
Inertia, 18
Infection, 25, 26, 59
  spread of, 45
Isometric muscle work, 40, 41

Joint limitation, 88, 89
  mobility, 58, 71, 93
  range, 24, 25, 26, 62, 90
Joints, ankle, 76, 107
  elbow, 99, 100
  hip, 92, 93, 96
  knee, 93, 96, 97, 106
  shoulder, 10, 70, 76, 100
  spine, 96, 101
Jumping, 117

Knee flexion, 41
Kneeling, 37
Kyphosis, 104

Laminectomy, 101
Lever, 9, 10, 11

Ligament, cruciate, 105
lateral of knee, 105
medial of knee, 105
rupture, 104, 105
strains, 104
Linen, 48, 56, 57
Liquids, 4
Lower motor neurone lesion, 71, 73, 77, 82
Lying float support, **34**, 38
half support, **35**
half support prone, **36**
half support side, **36**
head support, **36**
inclined support, **35**
support, **33**
support prone, **36**
support side, **36**

Mass, 4
Mass patterns, 38, 76, 83
Matter, 4, 14
Menisectomy, 97
Menstruation, 59
Metabolism, 22, 23
Moment of buoyancy, see Buoyancy
Moment of force, see Force
Movement, active, 75, 80, 82, 85
assisted, 10, 11, 24, 29, 30, 41
isolation of, 25
limitation of, 61
passive, 72, 73, 75, 76, 78, 80, 82, 83, 85
range of, 29, 40, 88
resisted, 10, 11, 15, 16, 19, 28, 29, 32, 33, 40, 41
voluntary, 71, 73, 74, 76, 81
Multiple sclerosis, 79
Muscle, power, 26, 58, 85, 88, 102
re-education, 11, 25, 71, 72, 79
rigidity, 81
strengthening, 25, 71, 93
weakness, 61, 74, 84, 88, 89, 91
Muscles, abdominal, 79
abductor of hip, 93, 95
abductor of shoulder, 78
extensor of back, 95, 109, 110

Muscles—*cont.*
extensor of elbow, 78, 80
extensor of hip, 30, 93
extensor of shoulder, 78
latissimus dorsi, 78, 79, 80
quadriceps, 63, 89, 96, 97, 102, 105, 106, 107
trunk, 80, 91

Neurological disorders, **71**
Neuropraxia, 84
Neurotmesis, 84
Normal (*see also* Refraction), 15, 16

Oedema, 75, 88, 89
Orthopaedic conditions, 88
Orthotolodine test, **54**
Osteo-arthritis, 58, **62**, 98
Osteotomy, **93**
Oxford scale, 72, 82

Pack, 22, 27, **28**
Paget's disease, 104
Pain, 24, 25, 58, 61, 75, 79, 84, 88, 89
Parallel bars, 55, 76, 78, 94
Paralysis, 71
Paraplegia, 27, 58, **77**, 101
Parkinson's disease, **81**
Pascal's Law, **11**
Peripheral arterial disease, 60
Peripheral nerve lesions, 72, **84**
Peripheral resistance, see Resistance
Polyneuritis, 58, **84**
Pool, construction, **49**
depth, **50**
graded, 43, **49**, 50, 51
raised, **49**
sunken, **49**
Positions, starting, **33**
Posture, 93, 113
Postural defects, 104
Poundal, **4**
Precautions, 23, 26
Pressure, 12, 25, 40
fluid, 11
Progression of exercise, see Exercise

Proprioceptive neuromuscular
    facilitation, 38, 91, 99

Quadricepsplasty 98

Range of movement, full, 73
    inner, 11
    outer, 11
Records, 45
Recreational activities, *see* Activi-
    ties
Re-education of balance, *see*
    Balance
Re-education of muscle, *see* Muscle
Reflection, 15
Refraction, 4, **15**, 43
Relaxation, 24, 25, 70, 80, 81, 88,
    90
Resistance, manual, 40
Resisted movement, *see* Move-
    ment
Respiratory rate, 22
Respiratory disease, 60
Rheumatoid arthritis, 27, 58, **64**
Rhythmical stabilizations, 63, 78,
    91, 94
Rigidity, 72
Rooms, changing, **48**
    linen, **57**
    rest, 48, 49, **56**
    utility, 48, 57
Rotator cuff lesions, 70

Scalds, 44
Scoliosis, 104
Sensory loss, 84
Shoes, **55**
Shortening, apparent, 89
    true, 89
Shower, 26, 27, 55, 57
Sidewalk, 53
Sitting, **36**
Skin, 26, 74, 85
Skin temperature, *see* Temperature
Solids, 4
Spasticity, 58, 72, 74, 75, 76, 79
Spinal fusion, 92, 103

Spondylolithesis, 92, 104
Spondylosis, 104
Standing, **36,** 117
    inclined, **37**
Starting positions, *see* Positions
State, change of, 4
Sticks, 8, 28, 55
Straps, 33, 34
Streamlined body, 18, 29, 31, 40
    flow, 16, **17,** 31
Steps, **52,** 77
Stretcher, 43, 64
Support, 24, 29, 31, 72
Surface tension, 4, **15**, 29
Sweat glands, 22
Swimming, 25, 42, 48, 64, 70, 77,
    79, 80, 82, 83, 84, 91, 95,
    96, 100, 101, 106, 110, 111,
    112
    underwater, 70, 104
Synovectomy, 92, 97
Synovitis, 105

Tables of exercises, 63, 64, 65, 66,
    69, 81, 86, 87, 93, 94, 95, 100,
    102, 103,
Temperature, 16, 22, 23, 26
    body, 21
    pool, 27, 53
    skin, 21, 23
    water, 21, 52
Tiles, non-slip, 42
Tinea capitis, 46
Tinea pedis, 26, **46,** 59
Treatment, length of, 21, 25, 27,
    75, 93
Trophic changes, 74, 85
Turbulence, 16, 18, 19, 20, 24, 29,
    40, 46, 78, 113
Turbulent flow, 16, **17,** 18

Unstreamlined body, 18, 29, 31
Untoward effects, *see* Effects
Upper motor neurone lesion, 71,
    72, 73, 77, 79
Upthrust, 6, 8, 11, 29

Velocity, critical, 17
Ventilation, 49
Viscosity, 4, **16**
Vital capacity, 12, 60, 68, 70, 77, 83, 104
Volume, 5
Voxan disinfectant, 47

Wake, 18, 40
Walking, 25, 26, 67, 94, 95, 101, 106, 107, 117

Walking—*cont.*
    re-education of, 76, 82, 93, 98, 103, 109, 110
Water, pH value, 53
    physical properties of, **4**
    pressure, 11, 12, 25, 75
Weight, **4,** 5, 6
    arm, 24, 29, 32, 33
    bearing, 88, 106
    relief, 11
    transference, 66, 76, 94, 106
Weightlessness, 12, 24, 58, 75
Wheelchair, 54